Parviz Kambin

ARTHROSCOPIC MICRODISCECTOMY

Minimal Intervention in Spinal Surgery

ARTHROSCOPIC MICRODISCECTOMY

Minimal Intervention in Spinal Surgery

edited by

Parviz Kambin, M. D.

The Graduate Hospital
Director, Disc Treatment and Research Center
Clinical Associate Professor
Department of Orthopaedic Surgery
University of Pennsylvania School of Medicine
Philadelphia

with 15 contributors

Urban & Schwarzenberg
Baltimore – Munich

Urban & Schwarzenberg, Inc.
7 E. Redwood Street
Baltimore, Maryland 21202
USA

Urban & Schwarzenberg GmbH
Landwehrstrasse 61
D-8000 München 2
West Germany

Notices

The Editors (or Authors) and the Publisher of this work have made every effort to ensure that the drug dosage schedules herein are accurate and in accord with the standards accepted at the time of publication. The reader is strongly advised, however, to check the product information sheet included in the package of each drug he or she plans to administer to be certain that changes have not been made in the recommended dose or in the contraindications for administration.

The Publishers have made an extensive effort to trace original copyright holders for permission to use borrowed material. If any have been overlooked, it will be corrected at the first reprint.

5	4	3	2	1
94	93	92	91	90

Library of Congress Cataloging-in-Publication Data

Arthroscopic microdiscectomy: Minimal intervention in spinal surgery
/ edited by Parviz Kambin ; with 15 contributors.
        p.   cm.
    Includes bibliographical references.
    ISBN 0-8067-1081-0
        1. Vertebrae, Lumbar--Surgery. 2. Discectomy. I. Kambin, Parviz.
    [DNLM: 1. Intervertebral Disk Displacement--Surgery. 2. Lumbar
Vertebrae--surgery.   WE 740 A787]
    RD771.I6A57   1991
    617.3'75059--dc20   90-12125
    DNLM/DLC   CIP
    for Library of Congress   Rev.

Sponsoring Editor: Charles W. Mitchell
Managing Editor: Kathleen C. Millet
Manuscript Editor: Andrea Clemente
Printer: Kösel, Kempten
ISBN 0-8067-1081-0   Baltimore

ISBN 3-541-71081-0   Munich

Dedicated to

My wife, Helen Perkinson Kambin, and all my children.
My late parents, Mr. and Mrs. S. A. Missaghian Shirazi.
Without their support and sacrifices this work would not have been possible.

Preface

The evergrowing cost of medical care and the socioeconomical demand for early recovery and mobilization dictate the need for medical parsimony and striving for the development of minimal invasive operative procedures that are effective and cost-efficient.

This text has been developed to provide the readers with both scientific and technical details of the percutaneous approach to the lumbar spine. The development and utilization of the percutaneous technique for the treatment of herniated lumbar discs have been slow but progressive. This course was intentionally chosen to ensure safety prior to its wide distribution.

The table of contents, index, and sections which include several chapters authored by various contributors should facilitate easy access and localization of the desired subjects. The contribution of various authorities on given subjects should provide the readers with a broad and unbiased knowledge of several surgical techniques.

Finally, I must express my appreciation to the distinguished scientists and physicians: Peter Wolf Ascher, John BianRosa, John Goode, Richard Guyer, Hans-Jörg Leu, Wesley Parke, Adam Schreiber, Harry Schwamm, J. A. N. Shepperd, George Teplick, and Robert Watkins for their kind support and contributions.

Parviz Kambin, M. D.

TABLE OF CONTENTS

CONTRIBUTORS

Peter W. Ascher, M. D.
Universitätsklinik für Neurochirurgie
Karl-Franzens-Universität
A-8036 Graz
Austria

John J. BianRosa, M. D.
The Graduate Hospital
Anesthesia Department
One Graduate Plaza, 2nd Floor
Clinical Associate Professor of Anesthesia
University of Pennsylvania School of Medicine
Philadelphia, PA 19146

John G. Goode, M. D.
The Graduate Hospital
Anesthesia Department
One Graduate Plaza, 2nd Floor
Clinical Assistant Professor of Anesthesia
University of Pennsylvania School of Medicine
Philadelphia, PA 19146

Richard D. Guyer, M. D.
Co-Director, Texas Pack Institute
301 West 15th Street
Plano, TX 75075
Associate Clinical Professor
Department of Orthopaedics
University of Texas Southwestern Medical
School
Dallas, TX 75222

Peter Holzer, M. D.
Universitätsklinik für Neurochirurgie
Karl-Franzens-Universität
A-8036 Graz
Austria

Parviz Kambin M. D.
The Graduate Hospital
Director, Disc Treatment and Research Center
2027 Pine Street
Clinical Associate Professor
Department of Orthopaedic Surgery
University of Pennsylvania School of Medicine
Philadelphia, PA 19103

Hans-Jörg Leu, M. D.
Attending Orthopaedic Surgeon
Balgrist Medical School
University of Zürich
Zürich, Switzerland

Wesley W. Parke, Ph. D.
Chairman, Department of Anatomy
University of South Dakota School of Medicine
Vermillion, SD 57069

Adam Schreiber, M. D.
Professor and Chairman
Department of Orthopaedic Surgery
Balgrist Medical School
University of Zürich
Zürich, Switzerland

Oskar Schröttner, M. D.
Universitätsklinik für Neurochirurgie
Karl-Franzens-Universität
A-8036 Graz
Austria

Harry A. Schwamm, M. D.
The Graduate Hospital
One Graduate Plaza
Suite 415, Pepper Pavilion
University of Pennsylvania School of Medicine
Philadelphia, PA 19146

J. A. N. Shepperd, M. D., F. R. C. S.
Royal East Sussex Hospital
Hastings Orthopaedic Center
Hastings, East Sussex, TN34 1ER
England

Bernd Sutter, M. D.
Universitätsklinik für Neurochirurgie
Karl-Franzens-Universität
A-8036 Graz
Austria

J. George Teplick, M. D.
Director, Division of General Diagnosis
Department of Diagnostic Radiology
Hahnemann University Hospital
Philadelphia, PA 19102

Hans Tritthart, M. D.
Universitätsklinik für Neurochirurgie
Karl-Franzens-Universität
A-8036 Graz
Austria

Robert G. Watkins, M. D.
501 East Hardy Street #200
Inglewood, CA
Associate Clinical Professor of Orthopaedic
Surgery
University of Southern California
Los Angeles, CA 90301

INTRODUCTION

History of Disc Surgery

Parviz Kambin

The review of the history of surgical treatment of herniated lumbar discs is not complete without a brief reference to the great investigators who contributed to the understanding of the anatomy of lumbar intervertebral disc and its surrounding neural structures, recognition of a protruded intervertebral disc, the objective findings associated with sciatic pain, and, finally, the connection between the protruded disc and sciatica. Although the normal anatomy of the intervertebral disc and its pathological state demonstrated by an abnormal protrusion was known for years, no causal connection between those and sciatic pain was drawn until the early 20th century.

The importance of the content of the spinal canal in the function of the limbs has been known for centuries. "The Dying Lioness," and Assyrian art work, dates back to 1650 B.C. and shows injury to the spine by an arrow associated with paralysis (Fig. 1). Hippocratic contribution (460–370 B.C.) to medicine includes the description of the sciatic nerve with no specific reference to its origin. After the 9th century, the Persian and Arabic knowledge of medicine was absorbed and

practiced in Europe. Until the mid 17th century, the medical curriculum of European universities was based on teaching and writings of Avicenna (980–1037 A.D.) a well known Persian physician and philosopher; particularly, when his "cannon of medicine" was translated to Latin. An early reference to the anatomy of the sciatic nerve and treatment of spine disorders is found in the Persian literature. A Persian minature (13) from about 1400 A.D. clearly demonstrates their depth of knowledge regarding the anatomy of the spine. It

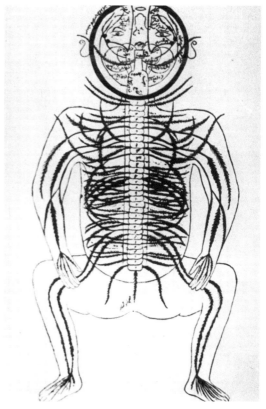

2 Persian miniature, from about 1400 A.D. (Reprinted with permission from McHenry-Garrison's *History of Neurology,* courtesy of Charles C Thomas, Publisher, Springfield, Il, 1969.)

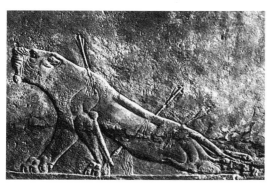

1 "The Dying Lioness" 1650 B.C. (Reprinted with permission from McHenry-Garrison's *History of Neurology,* courtesy of Charles C Thomas, Publisher, Springfield, Il, 1969.)

3

demonstrated the existence of 7 cervical, 12 thoracic, and 5 lumbar vertebrae and the origin of two components of the sciatic nerve from the lumbosacral segments (Fig. 2). There was no surgical treatment for back pain or sciatica. However; traction, manipulation therapy, and sedatives; namely, opium derivatives, were commonly used.

Most of the information regarding the anatomy and pathological changes of the intervertebral discs was gathered in the mid-19th century. Virchow (39), in 1857, described his autopsy findings of an intervertebral disc in a patient who expired following severe trauma. He called it a fractured disc and elaborated on its microscopic and gross appearance. Von Luschka (40), in 1858, found evidence of posterior disc protrusion of the intervertebral discs in cadavers in the course of routine autopsies. Kocher (18), in 1897, also reported traumatic injury to the intervertebral discs. In autopsy, he found posteriorly displaced discs at L1–L2 level; however, he did not relate his findings to the patient's predeath paralysis.

Schmorl (31), in 1926, on autopsy findings of 5,000 spines, reported approximately 15% posterior protrusion of the intervertebral discs in the spinal canal. He further contributed to the understanding of the anatomy of the intervertebral discs.

The term "sciatica" gained recognition as a clinical entity in the middle of the 18th century (1764) when Domenico Cotunio, an Italian physician, described its clinical manifestation. For a long time it was called Cotunio's disease. The signs and symptoms associated with sciatic pain were further defined by the contributions of Cotunio (1764) (5), Putti (1927) (29), Valleix (1941) (37), Lasègue (1864) (19), and Brissaud (3).

Goldthwait (14), in 1911, described the history and findings of a 39-year-old male who began to have low back pain, which was attributed to sacroiliac displacement. This patient underwent manipulation therapy for his sacroiliac disfunction; however, due to the development of paraparesis in the course of the above treatment, he was immobilized in a plaster cast and kept under observation. Six weeks later, the lumbar spine was explored, and extensive laminectomy from L1 to S2 was performed. No specific pathology was found at surgery except the narrowing of the canal at the lumbosacral articulation. Goldthwait concluded that the neurological deficit was due to detachment and outward protrusion of the annulus into the spinal canal, slippage of the articular process, and abnormality of the transverse process of the 5th lumbar vertebra.

In the early 20th century, laminectomy was being performed for the decompression of the spinal canal and, in some cases, for the relief of sciatic pain. Charles Elsberg (8), in 1913, reported 60 consecutive laminectomies performed at New York Neurological Institute and Mt. Sinai Hospital. In this paper, the author clearly describes the operative technique for laminectomy. Twenty-two of these operations were performed for tumors; 9 for section of posterior sensory fibers for the control of pain; 4 for inflammatory bone disease; 5 for old fractures; 2 had syringomyelia and hydromyelia; 1 for an intramedullary cyst; 1 for an aneurysm; 3 due to what was described as a peculiar disease of the nerve roots, and in 13 cases, no specific pathology was found.

Putti (29), in 1927, referred to the contribution of Sicard, who had performed laminectomy from the 3rd lumbar vertebra to the sacrum for relief of intractable sciatic pain. He also described the relief of pain for one of his own patients following a laminectomy and facetectomy for decompression of L5-S1 roots. Within a few years, the causal connection between the sciatic pain and protruded intervertebral disc was established. Elsberg (9, 10), in 1928, mentioned the chondroma of the vertebrae as causing compression of the equina. Stookey (35), in 1928, and Bucy (4), in 1930, also reported chondroma arising from the intervertebral disc, producing pressure on the neural structures. In 1929 Walter Dandy (7) from Johns Hopkins Hospital, reported two cases on whom he operated and removed "a completely detached fragment of cartilage from the intervertebral discs." Alajouanine (1), a neurologist residing in Paris in 1928, reported the extraction of a herniated disc in a 20-year-old female patient who demonstrated a motor deficit and had a positive Lipiodol myelography. Finally, the well-documented publication of the study by Mixter and Barr (22) in 1934, involving 19 patients, is credited for the popularization and acceptance of laminectomy for the decompression of the spinal canal and extraction of protruded lumbar discs.

The search for an alternative method of treatment for herniated lumbar discs began in the 1950's. Hult (16), in 1951, reported on his experience on anterolateral decompression of the herniated lumbar discs through a retroperitoneal approach Lewis Thomas (36) from New York University, under the sponsorship of The Commission on Acute Respiratory Disease, in 1956, reported the loss of rigidity and collapse of rabbit ears following the intravenous injection of crude papain. This condition reversed itself three to four days following the injection. Subsequently the introduction of chemonucleolysis by Lyman Smith (34) provided us with the concept that a herniated disc can be treated by an indirect approach without the need of visualization and extraction of the herniated site.

Love (20), in 1939, and Williams (41), in 1979, described their experiences in microlumbar discectomy which allows the entrance into the spinal canal though a small incision for the removal of disc fragments.

The percutaneous approach to the lumbar intervertebral discs represents a new concept in the treatment of protruded symptom-producing discs. In contrast to laminectomy or microlumbar discectomy, the spinal canal and its content is not violated in the course of this procedure.

A great attribution should be given to Valls et al. (38), Ottolenghi (27), and Craig (6), for their work and publications on the posterolateral approach to the spine. Although this procedure was principally described for biopsy purposes, the approach was later utilized for discography, chemonucleotherapy, and subsequently for the percutaneous lumbar discectomy. Ottolenghi's schemic drawing which demonstrates the proper positioning of the needle through the postereolateral approach has remained unchallenged.

Our experimental work with percutaneous lumbar discectomy began in 1973 (17). Our first patient was a 60-year-old male with right sciatica who had a disc protrusion at L3-4 and L4-5 levels. The L3-4 disc was excised following a laminectomy, while the L4-5 was decompressed and partially evacuated through a Craig cannula inserted dorsolaterally (Fig. 3). A 43-year-old female with

clinical and myelographic diagnosis of L4-5 disc herniation was exposed to a percutaneous lumbar discectomy in April of 1974; however, we were unable to reach the posterior fragments. This patient subsequently required a laminectomy for the removal of the sequestrated disc material.

In June of 1974, a 37-year-old male with persistent low back pain and left sciatica was admitted to the hospital. His myelogram showed disc herniations at L4-5 and L5-S1 levels. Both levels were explored surgically, and a large herniation at L5-S1 was found which was excised. The L4-5 disc was partially evacuated, utilizing a Craig cannula and small punch forceps. In February of 1974, a similar operation was performed on a 52-year-old male with right sciatic pain and myelographic evidence of disc herniation at both L3-4 and L4-5 levels. A large herniation at L4-5 was found which was extracted following a bilateral hemilaminectomy. The L3-4 level was decompressed and partially evacuated with a Craig cannula inserted through the percutaneous approach. Our subsequent experimental work in cadavers proved the safety of using forced suction in the intervertebral discs. From the pathological examination of the intervertebral discs in fresh cadavers, we learned the necessity of developing the technology which would allow us to reach posteriorly and evacuate

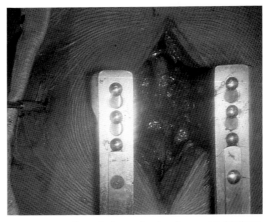

3 Interoperative photograph showing open laminectomy procedure combined with the introduction of working sheath into the intervertebral disc through a posterolateral approach for the purpose of decompression and evacuation.

the symptom producing fragments in certain patients.

In October of 1980, our preliminary experience and plans for the future treatment of patients with herniated lumbar discs by the percutaneous method was submitted to the Human Subject Committee of The Graduate Hospital, University of Pennsylvania, School of Medicine, for approval. The appropriate documentation for patient information and education was developed. Subsequently nine patients were treated under strict protocol by this method. The detailed clinical and myelographic findings, operative technique, and results were submitted to the *Journal of Clinical Orthopaedics and Related Research* on June 15, 1982, which was subsequently published (17). To the best of our knowledge, this report represented the first recognized publication of these findings in a medical journal of the world's literature. Dr. Hijikata (15) should be credited for his independent work on percutaneous nucleotomy in 1975 and his fine report in the *Journal of Toden Hospital* in Japan. This technique followed the principle of chemonucleolysis and was directed and designed for the extraction of the nucleus from the center of the intervertebral disc with a straight probe.

Friedman (12), utilizing Jacobson's operative technique in 1983, reported his experience with the introduction of a No. 40 French chest tube and speculum into the intervertebral discs through a 1-inch incision over the iliac crest. Due to the far lateral approach and the size of instruments, several complications have been encountered in the course of this operative procedure. The contribution of Schreiber and Suezawa (32), for biportal approach and discoscopy of the intervertebral disks and Monterio (23) for emphasis on a posterolateral hole decompression of the intervertebral disc deserve credit. Onik et al. (26), have introduced an automated instrument for nuclear evacuation following the principle of Hijikata's technique.

The names of the scientists, researchers, and clinicians who have contributed to the progress of disc surgery are too many to mention in this brief history. A great tribute should be given to Roentgen, a German physicist, for the discovery of the x-ray. Lipiodol myelography was introduced by Sicard and Forestier (33) which subsequently lead to the discovery of Metrizamide and other water-soluble radiopaque materials, and opened the path to the diagnosis and isolation of symptom-producing discs.

The contributions of Radon (30), Oldendorf (24, 25), Cromak, and Houndsfield, who subsequently, in 1979, shared a Nobel prize in medicine for the development of the CT scan, deserve recognition. The names of numerous scientists who have contributed to the development of MRI are too many to mention. Block (2) and Purcell (28), who shared a Nobel prize on this subject, should be remembered. The contribution of Farfan (11) for the understanding of the biomechanics of intervertebral discs and MacNab (21), in degenerative changes of intervertebral discs, deserve credit.

The scientists of our time, whose work keeps the flame of progress lit both in the field of disc surgery and the pathophysiology of the nerve root and the spinal nerve, are too many to mention and for this, I extend my apology.

References

1. Alajouanine, TH: From the presidential address by Professor Jean Cauchoix before Annual Meeting of the International Society for the Study of the Lumber Spine, San Francisco, Ca., June, 1978.

2. Block, F: Nuclear induction. *Physiol. Rev.* 70:460, 1946.

3. Brissaud: Quoted from Reynolds, F, and Katz, S: *Herniated Lumbar Intervertebral Disc.* American Academy of Orthopaedic Surgeons Symposium on the Spine. 84–96 CV Mosby Co., St. Louis, 1969.

4. Bucy, PC: Chondroma of intervertebral disc. J.A.M.A. 94:1552, 1930.

5. Cotunio, D: *De Ischiade Nervosa Canmentarius.* Simoncos Brothers, Naples, 1764.

6. Craig, FS: Vertebral body biopsy. *J. Bone Joint Surg.* 38A:93, 1956.

7. Dandy, WE: Loose cartilage from intervertebral disk simulating tumor of the spinal cord. *Arch. Surg.* 19:660, 1929.

8. Elsberg, CA: Experiences in spinal surgery: Observations upon 60 laminectomies for spinal disease. *Surg. Gynecol. Obstet.* 16:117, 1913.

9. Elsberg, CA: Diagnosis and treatment of surgical diseases of the spinal cord and its membranes. WB Saunders, Philadelphia, 1916.

10. Elsberg, CA: Extradural spinal tumors, primary, secondary, metastasis. *Surg. Gynecol. Obstet. 46:1, 1928.*

11. Farfan, HF: *Mechanical Disorders of the Low Back.* Lea & Febiger, Philadelphia, 1973.

12. Friedman, WA: Percutaneous discectomy: An alternative to chemonucleolysis. *J. Neurosurg.* 13:542, 1983.

13. *Garrison's History of Neurology.* Charles C Thomas, Springfield, IL, 1969.

14. Goldthwait, JE: The lumbosacral articulation: An explanation of many cases of "lumbago," "sciatica" and paraplegia. *Boston Med. Surg. J.* 164: 365, 1911.

15. Hijikata, SA: A method of percutaneous nuclear extraction. *J. Toden Hosp.* 5:39, 1975.

16. Hult, L: Retroperitoneal disc fenestration in low back pain and sciatica. *Acta Orthop. Scand.* 20:343, 1951.

17. Kambin, P, and Gellman, H: Percutaneous lateral discectomy of the lumbar spine: A preliminary report. *Clin. Orthop.* 174:127, 1983.

18. Kocher, T: Die Verletzungen der Wirbelsäule. Zugleich als Beitrag zur Physiologie des menschlichen Rückenmarks. *Mitt. Grenzgeb. Med. Chir.* 1:415, 1896.

19. Lasègue, CH: Considerations sur la sciatique. *Arch. Gen. Med.* 2:558, 1864.

20. Love, JG: Removal of protruded intervertebral discs without laminectomy. *Proc. Staff Meeting Mayo Clin.* 14:800, 1939.

21. MacNab, I: Disc degeneration and low back pain. *In Royal College of Physicians and Surgeons of Canada Annual Meeting Proceedings 3 and 4,* October, 1952.

22. Mixter, WJ, and Barr, JS: Rupture of the intervertebral disc with involvement of the spinal canal. *N. Engl. J. Med.* 211:210, 1934.

23. Monterio, A: Percutaneous Lumbar Discectomy, International Symposium, Graduate Hospital, University of Pennsylvania, March 1987.

24. Oldendorf, WH: Displaying the internal structural pattern of a complex object. *Ir. Trans. Bio-Med. Elect. BME.* 8:68, 1961.

25. Oldendorf, WH: *The Quest for an Image of the Brain.* Raven Press, New York, 1980.

26. Onik, G, Helms, C, Ginsberg, L, Hoaglund, T, and Morris, J: Percutaneous lumbar discectomy using a new aspiration probe. *A.J.N.R.* 6:290, 1985.

27. Ottolenghi CE: Vertebral body biopsy, aspiration biopsy. *J. Bone Joint Surg.* 37-A, June, 1955.

28. Purcell, EM, et al.: Resonance absorption by nuclear magnetic moments in a solid. *Physiol. Rev.* 69:37–38, 1946.

29. Putti, V: The Lady Jones lecture: Pathogenesis of sciatic pain. *Lancet* 2:53, 1927.

30. Radon: Quoted by Oldendorf, WH: *The Quest for an Image of the Brain.* Raven Press, New York, 1980.

31. Schmorl, G: Die pathologische Anatomie der Wirbelsäule. *Verh. Deutsch. Orthop. Gest.* 21:3, 1926.

32. Schreiber, A, and Suezawa, Y: Transdiscoscopic percutaneous nucleotomy in disc herniation. *Orthop. Rev.* 15:75, 1986.

33. Sicard JA, and Forestier, J: Méthode radiographique d'exploration de la cavité epidurale par le Lipiodal. *Rev. Neurol.* 37:1264, 1921.

34. Smith, L: Enzyme dissolution of the intervertebral disc. *Nature* 4887:198, 1963.

35. Stookey, B: Compression of the spinal cord due to ventral extradural cervical chondromas. *Arch. Neurol. Psychiatry* 20:275, 1928.

36. Thomas, L: Reversible collapse of rabbit ears after intravenous papain. *J. Exp. Med.* 104:245, 1956.

37. Valleix: Quoted from Reynolds, F, and Katz, S: Herniated Lumbar Intervertebral Disc. American Academy of Orthopaedic Surgeons Symposium on the Spine. CV Mosby, St. Louis, 1969.

38. Valls, J, Ottolenghi, CE, and Schajowicz, F: Aspiration biopsy in diagnosis of lesions of vertebral bodies. *J.A.M.A.* 136: 376, 1948.

39. Virchow, R: *Untersuchungen über die Entwickelung des Schädelgrundes*. G. Reimer, Berlin, 1857.

40. Von Luschka, H: *Die Gelenke des menschlichen Körpers*. IV. G Reimer, Berlin, 1858.

41. Williams, RW: Microsurgical lumbar discectomy. Report to American Association of Neurology and Surgery, 1975. *Neurosurgery* 4 (2):140, 1979.

SECTION I
ANATOMY AND PATHOLOGY

1 Clinical Anatomy of the Lower Lumbar Spine

Wesley W. Parke

Anatomical Relations of the Lower Lumbar Spinal Canal

The spinal canal is the continuous tube formed by the successive vertebral (spinal) foramina and their associated articulations. Although the neural contents of its cavity are effectively protected against all but severe traumatic pressures, it is rather ironic that it is the eventual degenerative derangements of the structure of the canal itself that provide the most common threat to its contained elements.

A constrictive alteration in the dimensions of the canal is termed a spinal stenosis (from the Greek, *stenos* = narrow). Its clinical severity is predicated on the original regional tolerances provided between the neural contents and the walls of the canal and the degree of encroachment caused by the pathological processes. Certain spinal regions, such as the lower cervical (22) and the lower lumbar, are dimensionally predisposed to stenotic syndromes whose variant symptomatology reflects the functions of the neural structures compressed.

Since the spinal canal below the second lumbar vertebra contains only the roots of the lumbosacral nerves, subjective evidence of a lower lumbar stenosis usually presents as some form of radiculopathy. In cross-section, the cavity of the lower lumbar canal appears as a triangle with a ventral base. The ventrolateral angles of this configuration form the lateral recesses which longitudinally accommodate the lumbosacral nerve roots in an already restricted space bounded by the subarticular part of the ligamentum flavum dorsally and the dorsolateral aspects of the disc ventrally. Unfortunately, the points of most frequent failure of the annulus in the degenerating lumbar disc are at the positions ventral to the lateral recesses on either side of the central strap of the posterior longitudinal ligament. At these points,

should the external rings of the failing annulus just be pushed dorsally by the herniating nucleus pulposus (bulging disc) or actually rupture to allow nucleus material to press against the dura (protruded nucleus), the end result is a lateral stenosis that may produce varying degrees of radiculopathy usually referable to the distribution of the spinal nerve exiting the foramen one vertebral level below the offending disc.

The schema presented in Figure 1-1, and the photographs in Figures 1-2 and 1-3, amply illus-

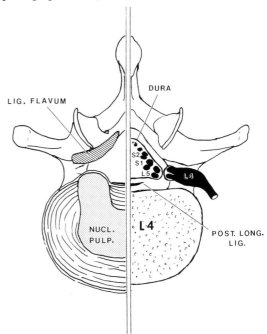

1-1 A schema illustrating a step-sectioned inferior aspect of a fourth lumbar vertebra showing the relations of the neural elements just inferior to the midsection of the vertebral body *(right side)* and the level of the L4-L5 disc *(left side)*. Note that the bulging disc would be inferior to the position of the L4 ganglion but would compress or alter the course of the L5 roots in the lateral recess. The lumbosacral roots maintain a fairly constant topography within the canal, with the lower sacral roots being more central and dorsal.

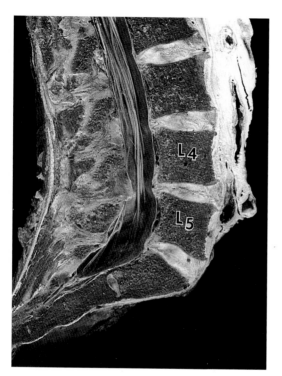

1-2 A nearly midsagittal section of a frozen lower lumbosacral spine from a 62-year-old male showing only the left side of the cauda equina. Note that the roots course in the lateral recesses between the discs and the subarticular ligamenta flava superior to their entrance into the thecal evaginations.

trate the vulnerability of the nerve roots in the lateral recesses. Figures 1-2 to 1-4 also reveal why the usual discogenic lateral stenosis does not compromise the spinal nerve of the same level. The dimensions of the lumbar intervertebral foramen are such that the exiting nerve roots are closely applied to the inferiomedial border of their respective pedicle and then turn lateral to exit through the superior half of the foramen. Since the disc lies ventral only to the inferior half of the foramen, the common type of dorsal encroachment misses its segmentally equivalent nerve but compromises the next most lateral nerve elements which, at this point, are the roots of the immediately inferior segmental nerve.

As can be seen in the sagittal section in Figure 1-2, the dura occupies most of the space in the spinal canal and provides a fluid-filled cavity that allows considerable motion to the contained root

elements. Although the position of the roots may initially appear to have a rather random arrangement, the roots are actually quite orderly in the manner in which they descend the canal as in Figure 1-1. The sagittal section (Fig 1-2) shows only the roots of the left side of the cauda equina where it may be discerned that their relative position is well controlled by their origins and exits. Those of the sacral nerves run in the more medial and dorsal positions, as they must be strung against the dorsum of the canal when they negotiate the directional change produced by the rather abrupt lordosis of the lumbosacral junction.

At the mid-L4 and L5 levels, this sagittal section illustrates, particularly with the ventral roots, how these structures enter an evagination of the dura that forms the thecal sheath. It may also be noted that, as these roots approach the level of their dural sheath exit, they occupy the narrow groove formed by the lateral recess. This space confines them between the bulge of the preceding disc and its dorsally related structures before they curve laterally to enter the dural theca and exit the canal through the next lower foramen. The photograph visually explains why a nerve root is usually affected by a dorsal protrusion of the disc that is one segmental level above the foramen of its exit from the spinal canal. By comparing this figure with the subsequent photograph (Fig. 1-3) and graphic schema (Fig. 1-4), a three-dimensional relationship of the spinal nerves, roots, and the dorsal root ganglia with their respective pedicles, thecal extensions, vessels, and attachments of the psoas muscles may be appreciated.

Figure 1-3 is a composite of frontal sections that were obtained by cutting a block of frozen lower lumbar vertebrae in 5-mm sections. As the sections were straight and vertical through the curvature of the lower lumbar lordosis, variant aspects of the contents of the lower three lumbar intervertebral foramen may be ascertained. The left side of the composite presents a plane ½ cm ventral to the surface as shown on the right side of the figure. It includes only the last three lumbar ventral roots, but as it retained the ventral dura, the actual levels of the discs are revealed (arrows), and positions of the L3, L4, and L5 dorsal root ganglia are better shown. The right side of the figure includes most of the dorsal roots and provides a better concept of

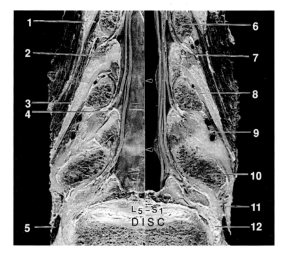

absorption of some of the ceretrospinal fluid (CSF) at this point. Just lateral to the ganglion, the musculocutaneous branch of the fourth lumbar artery, flanked by two veins, is evident.

In these frontal sections, the third lumbar nerve shows its oblique and caudally directed course between slips of origin of the psoas muscles that arise on the inferolateral aspects of the pedicles. This muscle also arises from the adjacent lateral surfaces of the discs and the inferioventral surfaces of the transverse processes. Of particular interest is the distribution of fat around and within the

1-3 Photographs of frontal sections from a lower lumbar spine of a 58-year-old male. The sections were cut at 5-mm intervals. The left side of the illustration shows the dural bulges indicating the levels of the third and fourth lumbar discs *(arrows)*, while the right side includes dorsal as well as ventral roots. The curve of the lumbar lordosis gives different section depths to each vertebral level. Note the relations of dorsal root ganglia and spinal nerves to ambient structures. *(1)* Slip of psoas muscle arising from external surface of pedicle. *(2)* Third lumbar dorsal root ganglion. *(3)* Ventral ramus of third lumbar spinal nerve. *(4)* Thecal sleeve of dura containing fourth lumbar nerve roots. *(5)* Iliolumbar vein. *(6)* Pedicle of third lumbar vertebra. *(7)* Musculocutaneous branch of third lumbar segmental artery. *(8)* Extension of intraforaminal fat that cushions spinal nerve. *(9)* Fourth lumbar segmental artery flanked by corresponding veins. *(10)* Pedicle of fifth lumbar vertebra. Note comparatively large size to buttress thrust of L5-S1 angulation. *(11)* Branches of the lumbar artery of the iliolumbar complex. *(12)* Fifth lumbar spinal nerve.

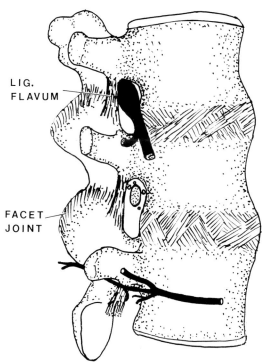

the root relationships to the discs one level above their foramen of exit.

Careful analysis of the structures shown in the above figure will reveal the relative length of the L4 thecal sheath (left side) that may be seen surrounding the last centimeter of the stump of its dorsal root and the termination of the ventral root. Note also the vascular relationships of this ganglion. Where the thecal sheath commences to expand over the ganglion, a complex vascular arrangement may be seen at its proximal pole. This is primarily a venous plexus that receives the radicular and medullary veins and assists in the

1-4 A schema of "generic" (no specific levels intended) lumbar vertebrae depicting the neural and vascular relations of the intervertebral foramina. The first level shows an intraforaminal dorsal root ganglion exiting the top half of the foramen. The second level shows the position of a sectioned ganglion relative to the three typical vertebromedullary branches of the segmental artery. The usual position of the sinuvertebral nerve *(solid black structure)* when entering the foramen is at the upper margin of the disc. Note that bulging of the disc would not usually spatially compromise the exiting neural elements. The third level indicates the usual position of the segmental artery and its branches relative to the pedicle, transverse process, and upper part of the intervertebral foramen.

intervertebral foramen. Seldom mentioned in detailed anatomical descriptions, this fat mass is often regarded as an adventitial filler of epidural and intervertebral spaces. However, a study of the various sections of these regions shows that this fat has a rather firm character and forms a mechanically supportive "bushing" for structures entering and leaving the spinal canal. A prominent extension of this fat body also follows the inferior and ventral surfaces of each lumbar nerve and is thus interposed between this structure and the external surfaces of the pendicle and vertebral body that define the inferior part of the intervertebral foramen. Its amelioration of the downward and ventral distraction that accompanies the spine and lower limb motions is obvious. The consistency and uniformity of this intervertebral fat mass indicate that it is not just another deposition of metabolical reserve tissue, but it is a definite anatomical structure with a biomechanical purpose.

The above discussion primarily pertains to the limited root involvement encountered with the relatively uncomplicated discogenic lateral stenosis that is amenable to percutaneous procedures. However, it must be kept in mind that disc degeneration is often only the first step in a sequence of degenerative events that often extends to the other components of the motion segment unit. Thus, multiple root involvement may signal more advanced conditions, such as a massive central disc herniation (cauda equina syndrome) or hypertrophic changes in the facet joints and ligamenta flava, often complicated by a spondylolisthesis (particularly at the L4-L5 level). These more extensive stenoses obviously require more aggressive decompressive approaches.

Lumbosacral Nerve Root Variations

In most instances of disc herniation, lumbosacral radicular symptoms will provide a fairly reliable indication of the vertebral level involved. However, a sufficient number of cases occur in which the neurological findings are ambiguous or frankly misleading, and additional diagnostic procedures should always be used to confirm the segmental level(s) of the lesioned disc(s).

There are a number of anatomical variations in the relations of the lumbosacral roots that may be responsible for inconclusive neurological indications. The most common would involve atypical origins or foraminal exits of individual lumbosacral roots. Although myelographic studies have indicated only a 4% incidence in such lumbosacral root anomalies, an anatomical study by Kadish and Simmons (9) has raised this figure to 14%, with the L5-S1 level being most commonly involved. Their observations provided four types of variations: *(a)* Intradural interconnections between roots at different levels; *(b)* Anomalous levels of origin of nerve roots; *(c)* Extradural connections between roots; *(d)* Extradural division of nerve roots.

An interesting source of confusing neurological findings may be due to the variant anatomy of the *furcal nerve*. This name has been applied to the fourth lumbar nerve as it exhibits a prominent bifurcation to contribute to both the lumbar plexus (femoral and obturator nn.), and the sacral plexus (lumbosacral trunk). However, Kikuchi et al. (11) have found that it is often indefinite in its intradural affinities, frequently exhibiting two dorsal root ganglia which have distinct root sources at the conus medullaris. They proposed that when symptoms indicate the involvement of two levels, suspicion should be directed to four possible causes: *(a)* Two roots may be compressed by a single lesion; *(b)* Two lesions may be present; *(c)* There may be an anomalous emergence of two roots through the same foramen; or *(d)* The peculiarly doubled components of the furcal nerve may exist.

Infrequently, variant "fixation" alters the expected sequences of nerve root exit. In a *prefixed* lumbosacral plexus, the furcal nerve (the division between the lumbar and sacral plexuses) exits through the third lumbar foramen, and the preceding and subsequent nerves exit one vertebral level higher than in the conventional distribution. Conversely, in the *postfixed* plexus, the furcal nerve exits the L5-S1 foramen, and the lumbosacral nerve sequence is then all one level lower than usually described (27).

Although Kadish and Simmons (19) noted that the existence of anomalous interconnections between nerve root levels dispels any notion of

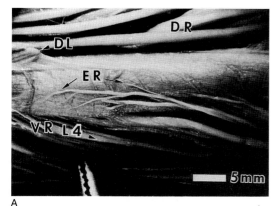

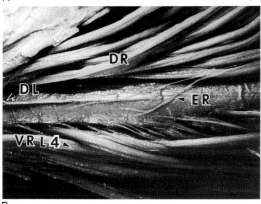

1-5 *(A)* A photograph of the lateral surface of a human conus medullaris showing the ectopic rootlets *(ER)* that receive axons from cells in the ventral horn nuclei. Note the origin of some fibers at the level of L4 motor nuclei that extend caudally to join the S1 root.
(B) A photomicrograph showing ectopic nerve rootlets *(ER)* passing dorsally to join a dorsal (sensory) nerve root. *DL* indicates the last denticulum of the deniculate ligament.

"absolute innervation," a more recent discovery has shown that there is a consistent system of intersegmental connections between the roots of the lumbosacral nerves. Parke and Watanabe (25) have described an epispinal system of motor axons that courses among the meningeal fibers of the conus medullaris and virtually ensheaths its ventral and lateral funiculi between the L2 and S2 levels. These nerve fibers apparently arise from motor neuron cells of the ventral horn gray matter and join spinal nerve roots caudal to their level of origin. In all the studied spinal cords, many of these axons comingled at the cord surface to form an irregular group of ectopic rootlets that could be

visually traced to join conventional spinal nerve roots at one to several segments inferior to their original segmental level (Figs. 1-5 and 1-6). On occasion, these ventral ectopic rootlets coursed dorsocaudally to join a dorsal (sensory) nerve root. Although the function and clinical significance of this epispinal system of axons are yet to be explained, they definitely demonstrate that a given segmental level of motor nerve cells may contribute fibers not only to an adjacent segment but also to nerve roots of multiple inferior levels.

An additional variant aspect of the lumbosacral nerve roots concerns the relative location of their dorsal root ganglia. Almost all anatomical illustrations will depict the lumbosacral dorsal root ganglia in an intraforaminal position with the central part of the ganglion lying between the adjacent pedicles. However, Hasue (Personal communication, 1989), by a method of nerve root infiltration (Kikuchi and Hasue, 12), has demonstrated that the lumbosacral dorsal root ganglia may also be positioned internal or external to their foramina. He designated the internal positions as *subarticular* or *sublaminar,* depending on their relation to these structures roofing the spinal canal, and found that approximately on-third of the L4 and L5 ganglia were in the subarticular position. It is obvious that if the ganglion is subarticular, it is in the lateral recess and subject to the direct consequences of a discogenic lateral spinal stenosis. When the ganglion is thus spatially compromised, there is no mystery about the source of the radicular pain; for it has been established that the ganglion is very mechanosensitive and will initiate nerve discharges under even slight external pressures.

The Sacroiliolumbar Arterial System

From the second thoracic to the fourth lumbar vertebra, the spine and its regionally related structures are supplied by pairs of segmental arteries that are direct branches of the aorta. However, since the aorta terminates in a bifurcation ventral to the fourth lumbar vertebral body, the vertebrae and the associated tissues caudal to this point must rely on an arterial complex derived mostly from the internal iliac (hypogastirc) arteries. Although

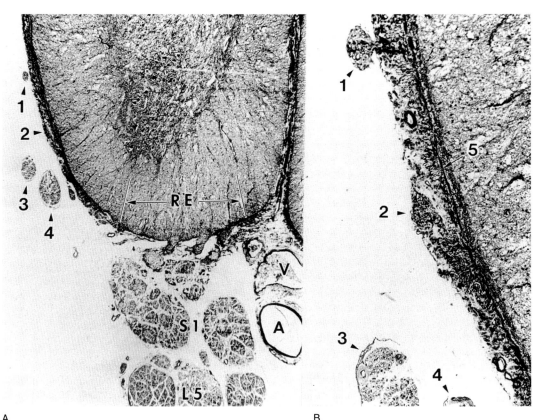

A

B

1-6 Photomicrographs of a 5-μm cross-section from the conus medullaris at the S1 level showing ectopic rootlets in various stages characteristic of their emergence from the ventrolateral surface of the cord. (Reprinted with permission from Parke, WW Watanabe, R: Lumbosacral intersegmental epispinal axons and ectopic ventral nerve rootlets. *J. Neurosurg.* 67:269–277, 1987.)
(A) Rootlets just appearing on the pial surface *(1,2)* will eventually join free rootlets *(3,4)* which have originated from higher levels. The conventional roots of L5 and S1 nerves have emerged from the typical zone of rootlet emergence *(RE)*. A and V are anterior spinal artery and vein. (× 33)
(B) A higher power photomicrograph of the preceding section showing greater detail of rootlet emergence. Note that the entire ventrolateral pia is intertwined with epispinal axons, of which only a few form ectopic rootlets. A dense circular band of pial straps *(5)* is characteristic of the region of the epispinal fibers. (×133)

this "sacroiliolumbar system," comprised of contributions from the fourth lumbar artery, the iliolumbar artery, and the middle and lateral sacral arteries, is of considerable functional significance, it has received only cursory mention in most anatomical texts and is almost never exposed in the routine dissections of medical anatomy instruction.

With the increasing use of percutaneous approaches to the lower lumbar discs, however, this infraaortric system of vessels has assumed a greater surgical significance, particularly due to the fact that, unlike the conventional segmental sup-

ply to the more superior vertebrae, its major components are longitudinally related to the dorsolateral surfaces of the discs most frequently involved in these procedures. Therefore, the conscientious operator should be aware of their presence, positions, and variability.

The Fourth Lumbar Arteries

The peculiarities of the sacroiliolumbar system of arteries may best be understood when compared with the pattern of distribution of the typical aortic

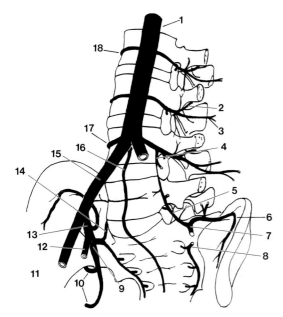

1-7 A graphic rendering of the distribution and major variations of the sacroiliolumbar system of arteries that supply the vertebrae and their associated structures inferior to the fourth lumbar vertebra. These patterns of the vessels were derived from radiographs of perinatal specimens and dissections of adults and then drawn against a tracing of the lumbosacral region taken from a left anterior oblique radiograph of an adult male. Note that the aorta lies to the left of center as it approaches the bifurcation ventral to the fourth lumbar vertebra. This schema shows the more frequent arrangement of the sacroiliolumbar system on the right side of the illustration where the iliolumbar vessel *(7)* has a single origin from the dorsum of the posterior division of the (removed) internal iliac artery. The left side shows the common variation where the iliac artery and the lumbar artery *(14)* are derived separately. The middle sacral artery *(16)* is in its typical position, and the anastomotic contribution from the fourth lumbar artery *(4)* shows its most frequent form. *(1)* Aorta. *(2)* Musculocutaneous branch of third lumbar artery. *(3)* Muscular branch to posterior abdominal wall. *(4)* Anastomotic contribution of the fourth lumbar artery to the sacroiliolumbar system. *(5)* Lumbar branch of iliolumbar artery. *(6)* Iliac branch of iliolumbar artery. *(7)* Iliolumbar artery. *(8)* Left lateral sacral artery. *(9)* Posterior division of internal iliac artery. *(10)* Superior and inferior gluteal arteries. *(11)* External iliac artery. *(12)* Anterior (visceral) division of internal iliac artery. *(13)* Internal iliac artery. *(14)* Variant origin of lumbar branch of iliolumbar artery from the lateral sacral artery. *(15)* Common iliac artery. *(16)* Middle sacral artery. *(17)* Left fourth lumbar segmental artery. *(18)* Left second lumbar segmental artery.

segmental branches. The ramifications of the fourth lumbar arteries were selected for this purpose, as they not only exemplify the conventional segmental distribution, but they are often involved in the nutrition of the next lower segments by variable contributions to the iliolumbar vessels.

Although extant texts fail to acknowledge some of the unusual features of the fourth lumbar arteries, the observations conducted for this writing have shown that these vessels often may be twice the caliber of their more cephalad homologues because of a greater muscular and intersegmental distribution.

As depicted in Figures 1-7 to 1-9, the distribution of the major ramifications is very similar to that of the thoracic segmental vessels with the exception of the additional branches that supply the psoas and quadratus lumborum muscles. Unfortunately, the drawing in Figure 1-9B separates the main segmental branch from the surface of the vertebral body for graphic clarity, but it must be realized that all the segmentals are immediately adherent to the surface of the anterior longitudinal ligament and the vertebral periosteum until they reach the region lateral to the intervertebral foramen. The lateral muscular branch (equivalent of the thoracic intercostals) may be quite large at the fourth lumbar where, in contrast to the other lumbar laterals, it passes anterior rather than posterior to the quadratus lumborum. It then continues to supply the lower posteriolateral abdominal wall as it courses superior to the crest of the ilium. As can be seen in Figure 1-6, it may be equivalent in size to the iliac branch of the iliolumbar artery, and its position superior to the crest would indicate that it is more liable to be encountered by percutaneous instrumentation than the latter vessel.

The dorsal musculotaneous branch of the fourth lumbar artery is equivalent in distribution to that of other thoracolumbar segmentals, as it usually displays a medial branch that supplies the external aspects of the facet joints and neural arch components and the transversospinal group of muscles, and a lateral branch to the transversocostal group of the erector spinae. The vertebromedullary (spinal) branches of the fourth lumbar artery are also similar to those of other segmentals. As can be seen in the radiograph of barium-injected vessels of a perinatal fourth lumbar vertebra (Fig. 1-9A),

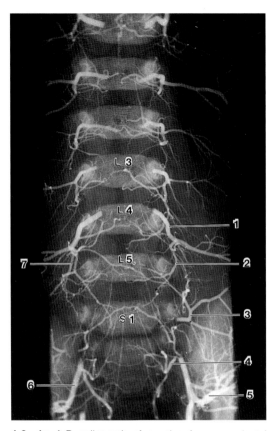

1-8 An A-P radiograph of a spine from a perinatal cadaver injected with barium sulfate. The aorta and common iliac vessels have been removed prior to radiography. This specimen was chosen because it showed considerable variation between the two sides of the sacroiliolumbar system. Note that on the right side of the illustration both a small lumbar branch and a descending branch *(2)* from the fourth lumbar artery enter the L5-S1 intervertebral foramen. On the left side, there is no lumbar branch, and a descending branch of the L4 artery supplies all of the vessels to the L5-S1 foramen. Also, the middle sacral artery is absent, and other branches of the system supply its domain. The radicular branches of the vertebromedullary vessels supply the distal radicular arteries and reveal the positions of the lower ends of the lumbosacral nerve roots. *(1)* Fourth lumbar artery. *(2)* Descending contribution of the fourth lumbar artery to the sacroiliolumbar system. *(3)* Iliolumbar artery. *(4)* Lateral sacral artery. *(5)* Superior gluteal artery. *(6)* Right posterior division of posterior iliac artery. *(7)* Derivatives of the fourth lumbar artery supplying areas normally supplied by the iliolumbar arteries.

they are a group of vessels of variable caliber that may generally be sorted into three divisions: *(a)* the ventral periosteal and osseous branches that supply the posterior longitudinal ligament, periosteum, and the cancellous bone of the vertebral body; *(b)* the radiculomedullary division that provides the irregularly located medullary arteries of the cord and the constant distal radicular arteries to all of the roots; and *(c)* the dorsal division which supplies fine articular branches to the deep aspects of the facet joints and the periosteum of the deep surfaces of the laminae and their associated ligaments. The first two divisions usually originate from a common branch of the segmental artery and enter the intervertebral foramen just rostral to their respective vertebral pedicle and ventral to the dorsal root ganglion, whereas the dorsal division arises from the musculocutaneous branch of the segmental artery and enters the foramen dorsal to the nerve components. All of the vertebromedullary branches may provide fine branches to the spinal dura.

The aortic segmental arteries course around their respective vertebral body at its narrowest circumference (Fig. 1-4) and thus come to be positioned almost equidistant between the adjacent discs. Hence, these parts of the arterial distribution are relatively safe from instrumentation properly positioned to enter the discs.

A major peculiarity of the fourth lumbar artery is its proclivity to provide a relatively large caudally directed intersegmental branch that arises near the level of the intervertebral foramen and becomes reciprocally involved with the lumbar branch of the iliolumbar artery. Thus, when this latter vessel is small or absent, the descending branch of the fourth lumbar artery may be sufficiently large to provide the predominant nutritional system to as many as two vertebral segments caudal to its origin (Figs. 1-7 and 1-8).

The Iliolumbar Artery

As opposed to the motly visceral distribution of the anterior division of the internal iliac (hypogastric) artery, the posterior division is essentially a somatic artery giving rise to gluteal, iliolumbar, and

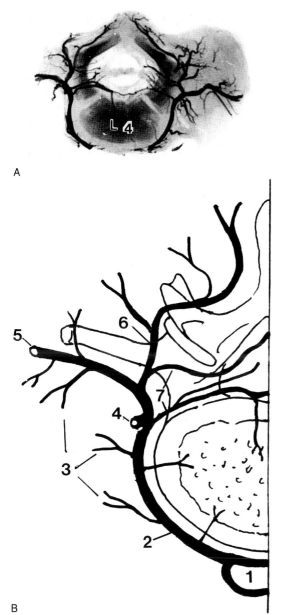

A

B

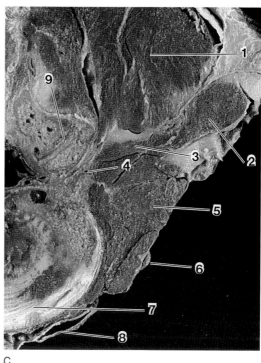

C

1-9 *(A)* A radiograph of a perinatal fourth lumbar vertebra after injection with barium sulfate to show the typical distribution of the lumbar segmental arteries.
(B) A graphic rendering of the distribution of the fourth lumbar segmental artery. *(1)* Aorta. *(2)* Fourth segmental artery. *(3)* Muscular branches to psoas and quadratus lumborum muscles. *(4)* Descending itersegmental contribution to sacroiliolumbar system. *(5)* Lateral muscular branch to posterior abdominal wall (corresponds to intercostal artery). *(6)* Musculocutaneous branch to dorsal spinal region and skin. *(7)* Vertebromedullary branches to internal aspects of spinal canal.
(C) A section through a frozen lumbar spine at the level of the L4-L5 disc. *(1)* Erector spinae muscle. *(2)* Crest of ilium. *(3)* Quadratus lumborum muscle. *(4)* Small descending branch of fourth lumbar artery. *(5)* Psoas muscle. *(6)* Tendon of psoas minor muscle. *(7)* Annulus. *(8)* Common iliac vein. *(9)* Facet joint.

lateral sacral branches. The iliolumbar artery most frequently is the first branch of this dorsal division, and it is directed dorsosuperiorly to pass close to the ventrolateral surface of the first sacral vertebral segment. It then passes superiorly dorsal to the obdurator nerve and ventral to the lumbosacral trunk. Its fairly consistent position between these two structures, as they pass over the L5-S1 disc to enter the pelvis, is well illustrated by the cross-section photograph in Figure 1-10B. Lateral to the inferior margin of the disc, the iliolumbar artery usually divides into a laterally directed iliac artery and an ascending lumbar artery. The first of these crosses the sacroiliac joint to reach the iliac

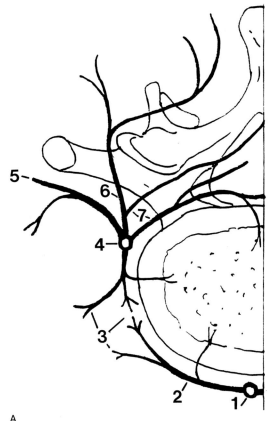

A

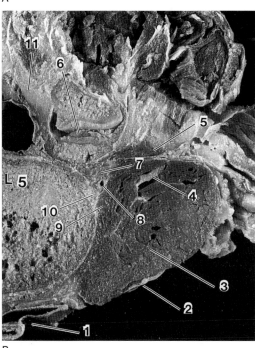

B

fossa of the pelvis where it courses inferior to the iliac crest and usually deep to the muscle to provide muscular branches to the iliacus muscle, articular twigs to the acetabulum, and eventually anastomoses with the deep circumflex branch of the femoral artery. The lumbar artery ascends posterolateral to the L5-S1 disc, still between the obdurator nerve and the lumbosacral trunk, to provide the vertebromedullary vessels to the L5-S1 intervertebral foramen (Figs. 1-7 and 1-10). In most cases, a branch of this vessels continues rostrally to anastomose with the descending branch of the fourth lumbar artery. The lumbar branch of the iliolumbar artery provides regional branches to the psoas and quadratus lumborum muscles but is reciprocal in this function to the relative size of the contributions of the descending fourth lumbar branch and/or the first lateral branches of the middle sacral artery (Figs. 1-7 and 1-8).

The Sacral Arteries

The Lateral Sacral Arteries

These vessels usually form the second branch of the dorsal division of the internal iliac arteries and course down the pars lateralis on each side of the sacrum. Opposite the sacral foramina they give off medial branches that dorsally enter the foramina, and, after providing the typical vertebromedullary derivatives, their dorsal muscular branches exit through the dorsal sacral foramina to supply the sacral origins of the erector spinae muscles.

1-10 *(A)* A schema of the vascularity derived from the sacroiliolumbar system at the middle of L5. *(1)* Middle sacral artery. *(2)* Segmental branch of middle sacral artery to fifth lumbar vertebra. *(3)* Anastomotic and muscular branches. *(4)* Descending branch of fourth lumbar and ascending branch of iliolumbar artery. *(5)* Lateral muscular branch. *(6)* Musculocutaneous branch of segmental artery. *(7)* Vertebromedullary arteries to L4-L5 intervertebral foramen.
(B) A photograph of a section through the fifth lumbar vertebra just above the disc. *(1)* Common iliac vein. *(2)* Psoas minor tendon. *(3)* Psoas major muscle. *(4)* Femoral nerve. *(5)* Quadratus lumborum muscle. *(6)* Facet joint. *(7)* Obturator nerve. *(8)* Lumbar branch of iliolumbar artery. *(9)* Sympathetic ganglion. *(10)* Lumbosacral trunk. *(11)* Ligamentum flavum.

The Middle Sacral Artery

This median unpaired vessel is the last branch of the aorta usually being derived from its dorsal median surface just above the carina of the bifurcation. It descends down the ventral surface of the anterior longitudinal ligament over the fourth and fifth lumbar bodies and down the ventral sacrum to terminate at the sacrococcygeal junction in a vascular glomus (sacrococcygeal body) in tailless mammals or continues ventral to the coccygeal (caudal) vertebrae in the tailed mammals as the caudal artery. In humans, this is a quite variable vessel, being totally absent in some cases or being replaced by a branch of one of the lateral sacrals. Where it is a significant component of the sacroiliolumbar system, its first lateral branches on the ventral surface of the fifth lumbar body may entirely replace this segment's contributions from the iliolumbar of fourth lumbar vessels and provide its osseous, muscular, and vertebromedullary requirements.

Where it is conspicuously present in the sacral region, it may also contribute a vertebromedullary branch to each anterior sacral foramen, and when totally absent, such as in Figure 1-8, these ventral sacral territories are provided with segmental medial branches from the lateral sacral arteries.

Functional Significance

The sacroiliolumbar system, despite its complexity and seemingly endless combinations of reciprocal substitutions, supplies the lower lumbosacral elements of the spine and the inferior half of the lumbosacral spinal nerve roots (cauda equina), as well as the back musculature inferior to the L4 level. It is also a major contributor to the vasa nervorum of the lumbosacral plexus. As demonstrated in the radiograph of Figure 1-8, the distal radicular arteries define the positions of the lumbosacral roots by their injected contrast medium. Although significant medullary branches to the spinal cord are seldom found below L4, they do occur, and, from the preceding descriptions, it is obvious why the ligation of both internal iliac arteries during radical cystoprostectomy has resulted in spinal cord ischemia (10).

Neuroanatomy of the Lower Lumbar Spine

The neural relations of the lower lumbar spine fall into two categories. The first concerns the normal and pathological intrinsic anatomy of the lumbosacral nerve roots and their relation to the segmental bone and connective tissues, while the second concerns the innervation of the motion segment structures themselves.

The Spinal Nerve Root: Its Intrinsic Anatomy and Vascular Supply

Although it has been generally recognized that much of lower back pain and sciatica results from compression or tension on the spinal nerve roots consequent to degenerative changes in the motion segment, the mechanisms by which the actual nerve discharge occurs were obscure. The nerve roots had long been regarded as histologically and nutritionally similar to peripheral nerves, and research on the latter was often uncritically extrapolated to apply to the nerve roots. The very long roots of the lumbosacral spinal nerves appeared to be particularly vulnerable with respect to their nutrition, as their vascularity could be supplied only from their ends without the access to frequent collateral support that is characteristic of peripheral nerves. It also appeared that the fine vascularity they possessed would be at risk from the repeated tension and relaxation resulting from the flexion and extension of the spine (Fig. 1-11). However, the reports of Parke et al. (23) and Parke and Watanabe (24) have shown that the roots receive an arterial supply from both ends (Figs. 1-12 and 1-13), and the existence of many redundant coils along the branches of the true radicular arteries ameliorates the stresses that would result from the interfascicular movements that would accompany the repeated stretch and relaxation (Fig. 1-14). A most significant finding was the occurrence of numerous and relatively large arteriovenous anastomoses throughout the length of the root. These vascular cross-connections apparently allow a blood flow to be maintained in sections of the root both above and below a point of compression (33). Of particular significance is the work of Rydevik and his associates (28) who,

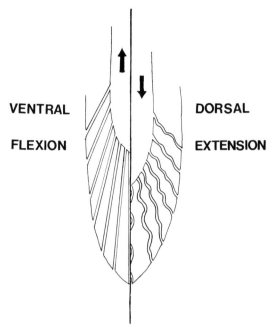

VENTRAL   DORSAL

FLEXION   EXTENSION

1-11 A schema indicating the cause of the interfascicular motion in the lumbosacral nerve roots and the need for interfascicular coils in the vasculature. (Modified from Breig, A, Marions, O: Biomechanics of the lumbosacral nerve roots. *Actaradiol.* 1Ö1141, 1963.)

using isotopically labeled methyl glucose demonstrated that approximately 50% of the root nutrition is derived from the ambient CSF; a fact that necessitates the gauze-like nature of the radicular pial sheath (Figs. 1-14B and 1-15).

A study of chronically compressed roots has indicated that the compressed segment is most likely metabolically deprived, and it has been strongly indicated that the pain is related to radicular ischemia as the reduction of oxygen intake in patients with neurogenic claudication exacerbates the symptoms (5). However, the studies on the intrinsic vasculature of the nerve root (24, 33) have suggested that the venous side of the system may be the more vulnerable to the spatial restrictions imposed by degenerative changes in dimensions of the spinal canal. The exacerbation of neurogenic pain in cases where spinal stenosis has been associated with venous hypertension has been recorded by clinical investigators. LaBan (14) noted that patients with diminished right heart compliance and spinal stenosis may eventually show neurogenic pain even in static or recumbent situations. This was attributed to an increased external pressure on the already sensitized roots by

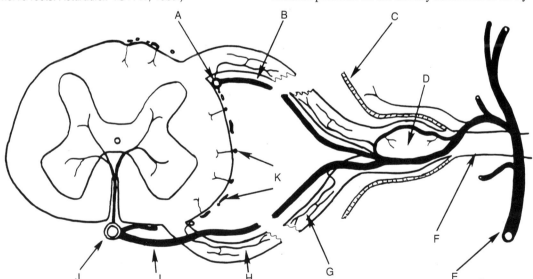

1-12 A schema illustrating all of the possible vascular relations of spinal nerve roots in which both medullary and spinal arteries are present. The break in the roots indicates that the schema applies to either the short cervical roots or the long lumbosacral elements of the cauda equina. (Reprinted with permission from Parke, WW, Gammel, K, Rothman, RH: Arterial vascularization of the cauda equina. *J. Bone Joint Surg.* 63A:53–62, 1981.) *(A)* Dorsolateral spinal artery. *(B)* Dorsal medullary artery. *(C)* Dura. *(D)* Dorsal root ganglion. *(E)* Segmental artery. *(F)* Spinal nerve. *(G)* Distal radicular artery(s). *(H)* Proximal radicular artery(s). *(I)* Ventral medullary artery. *(J)* Anterior spinal artery. *(K)* Vessels of vasa corona.

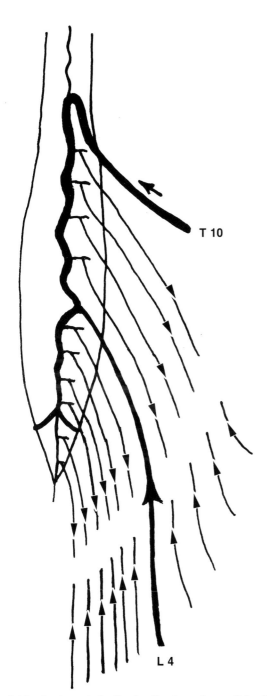

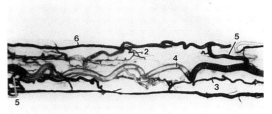

A

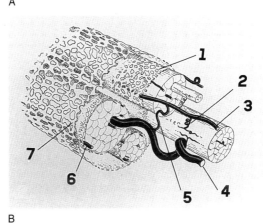

B

1-14 *(A)* A low-power (×20) transillumination photomicrograph of a midsection from part of an L4 nerve root that had been treated with hydrogen peroxide subsequent to vascular injection with latex-India ink but prior to clearing in a solution of tributyl-trycresyl phosphates. The peroxidases within the residual blood elements inflated the radicular veins *(4)* to provide a temporary contrast medium. Note the frequency of the large arteriovenous anastomoses *(5)* that permitted the latex-India ink to enter the veins.

(B) A graphic compilation showing the structure of a typical lumbosacral nerve root derived from data obtained by injection studies and scanning electron microscopy (see subsequent figure). The gauze-like pia-archnoid membranes permit the CSF to percolate into nerve tissues and assist metabolic support. Numbers in both *A* and *B* are common to equivalent structures. *(1)* Fascicular pia. *(2)* Inter- and intrafascicular arteries showing compensating coils to allow interfascicular movement. *(3)* Longitudinal radicular artery. *(4)* Large radicular vein (does not course with arteries). *(5)* Arteriovenous anastomosis. *(6)* Collateral radicular artery. *(7)* Gauze-like pia-arachnoid that permits percolation of CSF to assist in metabolic support.

1-13 A schema indicating the directions of normal blood flow in the cauda equina. Note that the anterior spinal artery of the lumbosacral part of the cord is supplied by medullary arteries and, in turn, supplies 75% of the cord substance and the upper parts of the cauda equina via the proximal radicular arteries. This accounts for the enlargement of the anterior spinal artery in the lumbosacral region.

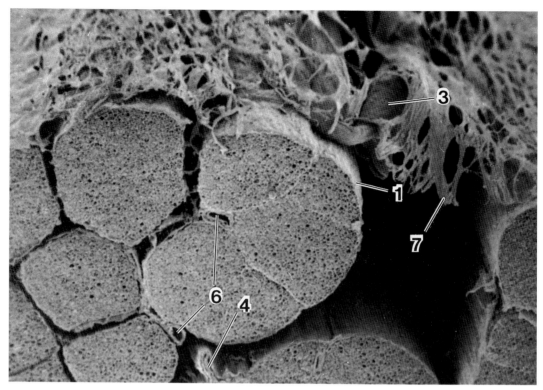

1-15 A scanning electron photomicrograph of a section of a proximal part of an L5 ventral nerve root. A gauze-like pia-arachnoid sheath is very evident. Numbers correspond to structures labeled in previous (Fig. 1-9) illustration. (×50.)

the engorgement of the epidural venous sinuses (Fig. 1-16). More recently, Madsen and Heros (15) showed that "arterialization" of spinal veins by abnormal arteriovenous shunts in the region of the conus medullaris exacerbated the neurogenic pain in patients with spinal stenosis. Their hypothesis suggested that a variable combination of increased mechanical constriction by dilated epidural veins and the direct increased resistance to the radicular circulation by the venous hypertension could contribute to the elicitation of the pain.

Thus, it appears that if the intrinsic circulation of the nerve root is impeded in either its arterial input or its venous outflow, the net effect is the same, namely, a neuroischemia of the compressed root segment(s) that may enhance the generation of ectopic nerve impulses.

A phenomenon that could be related to radicular venous stasis is the swelling of the disc-distorted

nerve root that Takata and associates (32) have well demonstrated in CT myelograms. This is difficult to explain since extravasated fluids in the root tissues should have free access to the surrounding cerebrospinal fluid. Nevertheless, the fluid balance of the root tissues appears to be altered, particularly in the segment proximal to the level of the offending disc, but the intricacies of the hemodynamic relationships responsible for this change remain unknown.

The role of the ubiquitous A-V anastomosis in the autoregulation of the intrinsic radicular vasculature also offers a fertile field for clinical investigations. As these vascular shunts are mostly without contractile elements but appear, instead, to control their lumina by the thickening response of an epithelioid endothelium, they probably react to chemical changes in the blood within their lumina and therefore offer an immediate local reflex to

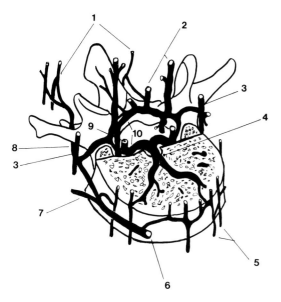

1-16 A schema showing the venous relations of a lumbar vertebra. Engorgement and a relative venous hypertension in the epidural vessels exacerbates neuroischemic conditions in the lumbosacral roots. *(1)* Dorsal external vertebral plexus. *(2)* Dorsal epidural plexus. *(3)* Ascending lumbar veins. *(4)* Basivertebral vein. *(5)* Ventral external vertebral plexus. *(6)* Lumbar segmental vein. *(7)* Muscular vein from posterior abdominal wall. *(8)* Musculocutaneous branch of external vertebral plexus. *(9)* Longitudinal channels (sinuses) of epidural plexus. *(10)* Circumferential channels (sinuses) of epidural plexus.

stimulated more serious inquiries. Over the past five decades, a number of investigations have attempted to delineate the origins, terminal ramifications, and nerve ending types of the sinuvertebral nerve, often with contradictory results. The more comprehensive works (2, 8, 18, 26, 31, 34) agree on the source and general composition of this nerve and describe it as variously branching from the distal pole of the dorsal root ganglion, the initial part of the spinal nerve, and/or the dorsal section of the gray autonomic communicating ramus. A multiple origin is common, especially in the lumbar region, and small autonomic branches often pursue a separate course and enter the intervertebral foramen independently. The largest component of the nerve passes through the anterosuperior part of the lumbar foramen cranial to the upper margin of the intervertebral disc and

alterations in the nerve root metabolism. Clinical evaluations of vasoactive compounds that may depress or excite nerve root irritability would be a rewarding area of study.

Innervation of the Spinal Motion Segment Connective Tissues

The distribution of medial branches of the dorsal ramus of the spinal nerve to the external periosteum, facet joints, and ligamentous connections of the neural arches, and the general ramification of the "recurrent" sinuvertebral nerve (nerve of Luschka, Basel Nomina Anatomica) to structures related to the spinal canal have been known for over a century. However, it was the recognition that degenerative disease of the intervertebral disc was a major cause of low back pain that has

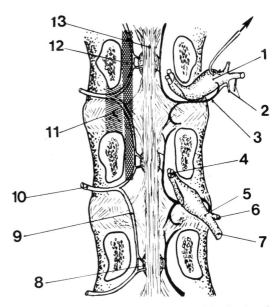

1-17 A schema showing the sources and distribution of the sinuvertebral nerves and the arteries serving the vertebrae and their associated connective tissues. *(1)* Dorsal root ganglion (retracted). *(2)* Rami communicantes of sympathetic chain. *(3)* Sinuvertebral nerve. *(4)* Lumbosacral spinal nerve roots. *(5)* Spinal nerve. *(6)* Dorsal primary ramus of spinal nerve. *(7)* Ventral primary ramus of spinal nerve. *(8)* Basivertebral sinus. *(9)* Descending branch of ventral vertebromedullary artery. *(10)* Ventral vertebromedullary artery. *(11)* Intraforaminal space. *(12)* Lateral recess. *(13)* Central strap of posterior longitudinal ligament.

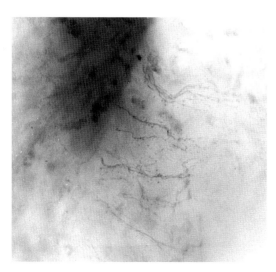

1-18 A microphotograph of the fine nerve endings in the lateral expansion of the posterior longitudinal ligament covering the dorsolateral surface of a dog lumbar disc. These nerve endings are believed to be nociceptive. Supravitally stained with methylene blue (Dogiel method) ($\times$ 300).

courses superomedially toward the posterior longitudinal ligament. As it approaches the ligament, it divides into superiorly and inferiorly directed rami which, in turn, provide numerous finer branches to the regional tissues (Figs. 1-17 and 1-18).

In illustrations based on dissections, Bogduk and Twomey (2) and Parke et al. (20) show that each nerve supplies at least two intervertebral discs. The inferiorly directed branch ramifies over the dorsum of the disc at the level of entry, while the longer superior branch courses along the lateral margin of the posterior longitudinal ligament to reach the disc of the next superior level. Contralateral overlap in the distribution of these nerves has been indicated, and an even greater multisegmental range in the distribution of the spinal dural branches has been reported by Kimmel (13). Thus, a basis for the poor pain localization of an offending disc may be related to the rather generous distribution of a single sinuvertebral nerve.

The posterior longitudinal ligament is highly innervated with both complex encapsulated nerve endings and numerous low-myelinated free nerve endings, but few investigators emphasize the fact that the lateral expansion of the posterior longitudinal ligament extends laterally through the intervertebral foramen and covers all of the dorsal and most of the dorsolateral aspects of the disc. Undoubtedly, the elevation of this thin, highly innervated strap of connective tissue may provide a significant component of the low back pain in acute disc protrusions.

The probable range of the diverse functions of the sinuvertebral nerve may be indicated by the analysis of its cross-sectional composition. Stained preparations taken from a section near the nerve origin showed many small myelinated fibers, but some myelin sheaths were in excess of 10 μm in diameter (26). There is little doubt that many of the smaller fibers are postganglionic efferents from the thoracolumbar autonomic ganglia that mediate the smooth muscle control of the various vascular elements within the spinal canal, and a number of the larger fibers are involved in proprioceptive functions. Concerning the latter, Hirsch and Schajowicz (8) and Parke (21) have found numerous complex encapsulated nerve endings in the posterior longitudinal ligament, and it is assumed that these may be associated with the larger myelinated fibers whose postganglionic axons enter the cord to mediate postural reflexes, since similar fibers in the cervical region of cats have been shown to be important in tonic neck reflexes (17).

It appears, however, that the smaller fibers which make up the greater bulk of the sinuvertebral nerve are afferents associated with the simple, nonencapsulated or "free" nerve endings that are generally regarded as nociceptive (Fig. 1-18).

That the sinuvertebral nerve carries pain fibers has been amply demonstrated by both clinical and laboratory experimentation. Direct stimulation on tissues known to be served by the nerve have been shown to elicit back pain in humans, and Petersen et al. (26) have shown that stimulation of these tissues in decerebrate cats has resulted in blood pressure and respiratory changes similar to those elicited by noxious stimuli to known pain receptors in other areas of the body. The essential question remaining then is in what components of the spinal motion segment are located the nociceptors responsible for the so-called discogenic pain?

There exists a major disagreement as to whether

the annulus itself is innervated, and if so, how extensively. The classic work of Hirsch and associates (7) claims that nerve endings may be demonstrated only in the dorsal aspect of the most superficial layer of the annulus and presumably from branches of the same nerve fibers that innervate the posterior longitudinal ligament.

Petersen et al. (26), Stilwell (31) and Parke (21) have also failed to demonstrate nerve endings in the annulus, and Parke believes that some reports of nerve endings in the superficial dorsal and dorsolateral aspects of the annulus may have resulted from including part of the unrecognized lateral expansion of the posterior longitudinal ligament in the analyzed sample. In all cases it is agreed that the connective tissue structures intimately related to the disc show a profusion of nerve endings which are most likely disrupted or stretched in deformations occurring at the surface of a pathological disc.

Hirsch and Schajowicz (8) noted that pressure on the normal disc does not cause pain, but an equivalent pressure on a degenerating disc produces back pain. Their conclusion postulated that the fissuring of the pathological disc permitted the invasion of granulation tissue that was followed by an ingrowth of nociceptive fibers into these metaplastic regions. Their opinion received later support in the excellent review of the literature and investigation by Shinohara (29) where he also claims that the degenerative fissures are invaded by fibroblastic tissue that subsequently receives an ingrowth of nerve endings. However, this concept has recently fallen into disfavor as Malinsky (16), Bogduk et al. (3, 4), and Yoshizawa et al. (35) have published accounts demonstrating nerve endings in the external one-third of the annulus.

The fibrous capsule as well as the synovial folds of the lumbar facet joints are well-innervated (6, 19, 31). The innervation of an arthritic facet joint may produce low back pain in conjunction with, or independent of, disc pathology at the same level.

The major descriptions of the distributions of the sinuvertebral nerve show that the bulk of the meningeal fibers enter the dura at its ventral surface where it approximates the posterior longitudinal ligament and the dorsum of discs and vertebral bodies. Since the dorsal and lateral dural surfaces are amply spaced from the corresponding walls of the spinal canal, perhaps there has been a general impression that the ventral dural surface also lacks intimate contact with the ventral wall of the spinal canal, and graphic depictions of the cross-sectional relations often give that impression. However, Parke (21) has observed that the ventral lower lumbar dura is often fixed to the ventral canal surface by numerous connective tissue fibers and most firmly fixed at the margins of the L2 to L5 discs. These adhesions are not to be confused with the ligaments of Hofmann (30), which are obliquely positioned by the developmental craniad traction of the dura and its contents. The above observation is supported by a series of dissections by Blikra (1) who was seeking a rationale for lower lumbar intradural disc protrusions. His analysis showed that the dura may, in some cases, be sufficiently fixed to the ventral surface of the canal, particularly at the L4-L5 level, that the protruding nucleus material can actually rupture the ventral dura. Given that these fibrous attachments may also conduct many meningeal nerve branches, the elevation of this area of the ventral dura by the herniating nucleus pulposus, on the basis of anatomical evidence and the conspicuous indentation of the dura often seen in myelograms, should be a significant pain-producing event.

Unfortunately, the actual pain, though mechanically caused, is a subjective phenomenon, and clinical observation is needed to confirm the occurrence. It is known that the conscious percutaneous discectomy patient may comment on the relief of pain, presumably due to the relief of intradiscal pressure, at the moment the annulus is fenestrated. This, however, does not necessarily indicate that the pain is only from intradiscal nerve endings, but rather that the pain-producing distortions, be they in the annulus or in the adjacently stressed structures, have been rather suddenly relieved.

It is very pertinent here to note that Dr. Vert Mooney (18), in his presidential address to The International Society for The Study of The Lumbar Spine, reviewed much of the current knowledge relevant to the production of low back pain and concluded that though the disc may be the primary source of the production of pain, the mechanisms by which the pain is produced are still uncertain, and much basic science and clinical investigation are needed in this area.

References

1. Blikra, G: Intradural herniated lumbar disc. *J. Neurosurg.* 31:676–679, 1969.

2. Bogduk, N, Twomey, LT: *Clinical Anatomy of The Lumbar Spine.* Churchill Livingstone, Melbourne, 1987.

3. Bogduk, N, Tynan, W, Wilson, AS: The nerve supply to the human lumbar intervertebral discs. *J. Anat.* 132:39–56, 1981.

4. Bogduk, N, Windsor, M, Inglis, A: The innervation of the cervical intervertebral discs. *Spine* 13 (1):2–8, 1988.

5. Evans, JG: Neurogenic intermittent claudication. *Br. Med. J.* 2:985–987, 1964.

6. Giles, LGF, Taylor, Jr: Innervation of lumbar zygapophyseal joint synovial folds. *Acta Orthop. Scand.* 58: 43–46, 1987.

7. Hirsch, C, Inglemark, B-E, Miller, M: The anatomical basis for low back pain. *Acta Orthop. Scand.* 33: 1–17, 1963.

8. Hirsch, C, Schajowicz, F: Studies on the structural changes in the annulus fibrosus. *Acta Orthop. Scand.* 22:184–231, 1953.

9. Kadish, LJ, Simmons, EH: Anomalies of the lumbosacral nerve roots. *J. Bone Joint Surg.* 66-B:411–416, 1984.

10. Kaisary, AV, Smith, P: Spinal cord ischemia after ligation of both internal iliac arteries during radical cystoprostectomy. *Urology* 25: 395–397, 1985.

11. Kikuchi, S, Hasue, M: Anatomic features of the furcal nerve and its clinical significance. *Spine* 11:1002–1007, 1986.

12. Kikuchi, S, Hasue M: Combined contrast studies in lumbar spine diseases. *Spine* 13:1327–1331, 1988.

13. Kimmel, DL: Innervation of spinal dura mater of the posterior cranial fossa. *Neurology (Minneap.)* 11:800–809, 1986.

14. LaBan, MM: "Vespers curse" night pain – the bane of Hypnos. *Arch. Phys. Med. Rehabil.* 65:501–504, 1984.

15. Madsen, JR, Heros, RC: Spinal arteriovenous malformations and neurogenic claudication. *J Neurosurg.* 57:793–797, 1988.

16. Malinsky, J: The ontogenetic development of nerve terminations in the intervertebral discs of man. *Acta Anat. (Basel)* 38:96–113, 1959.

17. McCouch, GP, During, ID, Ling, TH: Location of receptors for tonic reflexes. *J. Neurophysiol.* 14:191–195, 1951.

18. Mooney, V: Where is the pain coming from? *Spine* 12(8):754–759, 1987.

19. Nade, S, Bell, S, Wyke, BD: The innervation of the lumbar spine joints and its significance. *J Bone Joint Surg* 62-B:225–261, 1980.

20. Parke WW: Applied anatomy of the spine. Rothman RH and Simeone FA (eds.): *In The Spine,* ed 2, vol 1, ch 2. W.B. Saunders, Philadelphia, 1982.

21. Parke, WW: Paper delivered at the international Symposium on Percutaneous Lumbar Discectomy, Graduate Hospital, Philadelphia, Nov. 6-7, 1987.

22. Parke, WW: Correlative anatomy of cervical spondylotic myelopathy. *Spine* 13: 831–837, 1988.

23. Parke, WW, Gammel, K, Rothman RH: Arterial vascularization of the cauda equina. *J. Bone Joint Surg.* 63A: 53–62, 1981.

24. Parke, WW, Watanabe, R: The intrinsic vasculature of the lumbosacral spinal nerve roots. *Spine* 19:508–515, 1985.

25. Parke, WW, Watanabe, R: Lumbosacral intersegmental epispinal axons and ectopic ventral nerve rootlets. *J. Neurosurg.* 67:269–277, 1987.

26. Petersen, HE, Blunck, CFJ, Gardner, E: The anatomy of the lumbosacral posterior rami and meningeal branches of spinal nerves (sinuvertebral nerves). *J. Bone Joint Surg.* 38A:377–391, 1956.

27. Piasecka-Kacperska, K, Gladykowska-Rzeczycka, J: The sacral plexus in primates. *Folia Morphol. (Warsz.)* 31: 21–31, 1972.

28. Rydevik, B, Holm, S, Brown, MD: Nutrition of spinal nerve roots: The role of diffusion from the cerebrospinal fluid. *Transactions of the 30th Annual Meeting of the Orthopaedic Research Society,* vol 9, p 276. Orthopaedic Research Society, Atlanta, Feb. 7–9, 1984.

29. Shinohara, H: A study on lumbar disc lesions: Significance of free nerve endings in lumbar discs. *J. Jpn. Orthop. Assoc.* 44(8):553–570, 1970.

30. Spencer, DL, Irwin, GS, Miller, JAA: Anatomy and significance of fixation of the lumbosacral nerve roots in sciatica. *Spine* 8:672–679, 1983.

31. Stilwell, DL: The nerve supply of the vertebral column and its associated structures in the monkey. *Anat. Rec.* 125:139–169, 1956.

32. Takata, K, Inoue, S, Takahashi, K, Ohtsuka Y: Swelling of the cauda equina in patients who have herniation of a lumbar disc. *J. Bone Joint Surg.* 70-A:361–368, 1988.

33. Watanabe, R, Parke, WW: The vascular and neural pathology of lumbosacral spinal stenosis. *J. Neurosurg.* 65:64–70, 1986.

34. Wiberg, G: Back pain in relation to the nerve supply of the intervertebral disc. *Acta Orthop. Scand.* 19:211–221, 1949.

35. Yoshizawa, H, O'Brien, JP, Thomas-Smith, W, Trumper, M: The neuropathology of intervertebral discs removed for low-back pain. *J. Pathol.* 132:95–104, 1980.

2 Pathophysiology of Normal and Degenerated Intervertebral Discs

Harry A. Schwamm

The intervertebral disc is part of the mesenchymal system and arises from totipotential mesenchymal cells, as does all skeletal tissue. The "field" determines the activity of the mesenchymal cell.

Such an activity will determine which cell becomes an intervertebral disc and which one will form a cartilage anlage of the skeleton with the ultimate transformation into bone. This capability of all of these tissues to modulate within certain confines is maintained throughout life and certainly is demonstrable in the degenerating discs. This field differentiation is seen in the fetus or at the embryonic stage. So one can identify cells ultimately forming the annulus, others forming the intervertebral disc, the cartilage plate at either end of the disc, and ultimately the bony structure.

One does not see blood vessels in an intervertebral disc of adults, except under pathological conditions, but in the fetus the cartilage canals contain blood vessels, and nutrition of cartilage is always through diffusion from the cartilage canals. The next step in the development of the vertebral body and intervertebral disc follows the way any cartilage model skeleton is formed, in that the cartilage transforms itself, calcifies, and first becomes a matrix-containing cartilage body with calcification and ultimately transforms itself into bone. This process is essentially similar to that which is seen in a growth plate. The primary trabeculae and bone marrow spaces are created, thus providing adequate locomotor stability and necessary spaces for the marrow activity.

A slow but progressive transformation of cartilage to bone occurs. At the surface of the intervertebral disc a subchondral plate is formed, above it a definitive cartilage layer, and in-between the cartilage layers of two successive vertebral bodies; the fiber structure becomes the intervertebral disc. In a young child, the nucleus pulposus, which is so formed, exhibits a cellular structure, and as the child grows, this cellular fiber structure is capable of regeneration in order to keep up with structural demands. As soon as the maturity of the skeleton is developed, the fiber structure loses its prominent nuclear component, the cartilage tends to disappear, and, thus, all we have left in the adult is a bony plate and the relatively acellular intervertebral disc.

In a child of about three or four years of age, a clearly definable annulus and transitional zone between the annulus, nucleus pulposus, cartilage, and underlying subchondral plate is observed (Fig. 2-1). The nucleus has a soft and somewhat edematous cellular tissue, as compared to the denser fiber structure of the annulus fibrosis. Such a distinction is not seen in the adult life. The annulus of the adult consists of heavily collagenized connective tissue fibers inserting into adjacent bony structures of the vertebral body, similar to Sharpey fiber insertion at any other site.

In the adult, the fibers of the nucleus pulposus undergo normal aging processes, which start relatively early in life (age 35). Clefts begin to appear in the nucleus pulposus (Fig. 2-2) as the first sign of aging. With the progression of age, the nuclear clefts become larger and are associated with thickening, irregularity, and, finally, transverse and circumferential tearing of the annular fibers.

With the advancement of aging and the development of osteoporosis associated with the reduction of thickness and instability of the subchondral plate, small microfractures may cause the herniation of the nuclear material into the vertebral body, thus creating a Schmorl's node.

In cases of protrusion of the disc through or beyond the annulus fibers, there is an attempt at regeneration. Morphologically, this is characterized by metaplasia of the disc material into cartilaginous clusters. One sees regenerative clusters of cartilage cells within the disc (Figs. 2-3 and 2-4). Occasionally, this cartilage calcifies and reduces the resilience of the disc even further.

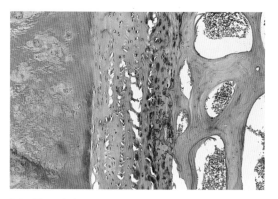

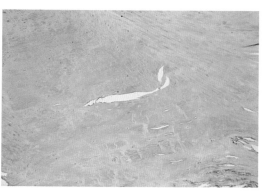

2-1 The relationship between mature disc material, cartilage, and the underlying subchondral plate is shown. Note the sharp demarcation between the intervertebral disc and cartilage in this young individual.

2-2 Early cleft formation in a degenerating disc. With age the clefts become more prominent.

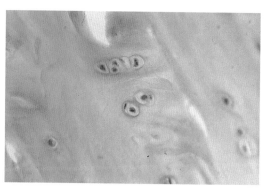

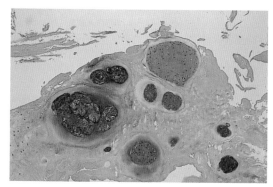

2-3 Cartilaginous metaplasia is seen in the extracted nuclear tissue for the treatment of herniated lumbar discs. Note the chondroid nuclei associated with clefts.

2-4 Prominent chondroid metaplasia with clusters of regenerating cartilage cells of a degenerated herniated disc, mimicking a cartilaginous neoplasm.

SECTION II
IMAGING

3 The Extruded Disc Fragment: Imaging Modalities

J. George Teplick

The Lumbar Spine: The Extruded Fragment

The detection of a fragment of a herniated disc is of considerable clinical importance. If a fragment is sequestered well above or below the annulus, the surgeon must be aware of its existence and exact location. Without this knowledge, the herniation may be removed at surgery, but the sequestered fragment may be overlooked. If the fragment is lying at the annulus level but is not recognized as a free fragment with computed tomography (CT) or magnetic resonance imaging (MRI), therapeutic techniques such as chemical nucleolysis or percutaneous discectomy will be ineffective. It might also be helpful to recognize when a herniation is extruded in situ, since this type may also not respond well to percutaneous discectomy. Extrusion, which refers to extension of a herniation posterior to a ruptured posterior longitudinal ligament, can sometimes be recognized or suspected if the herniation has an irregular or fuzzy posterior border or edge. The smooth posterior border of a herniation is mainly due to an intact posterior longitudinal ligament.

Figures 3-1A to E are line drawings of the cross-sectional appearance of a normal annulus (Fig. 3-1A), of a simple herniation (Fig. 3-1B), of an extruded herniation (Fig. 3-1C), of a fragment at the annulus level (Fig. 3-1D), and of a sequestered fragment (Figs. 3-1E1 to 3-1E2). These line drawings correspond to CT axial sections.

In the normal annulus at Figure 3-1A the intact nucleus pulposus remains confined to the mid-portion of the intervertebral disc; the annulus, its fibers, and the posterior longitudinal ligament (PLL) are intact. In Figure 3-1B, a simple herniation, the nuclear material has spread through the annulus, disrupting its posterior fibers and protruding into the canal. The PLL is still intact and makes up the posterior border of the herniation. In

Figure 3-1C, the nuclear material has broken through the PLL and is an extruded herniation. In Figure 3-1D, a piece of the extruded herniation has broken away from the main herniation and now is a free fragment but remains at the annulus level. In 3-1E1, there is a small extruded herniation; in Figure 3-1E2, at a level 1.0 to 1.5 cm below (or above) the annulus level, a free fragment is pressing into the right side of the thecal sac. Usually this sequestered fragment must be identified and surgically removed to attain successful treatment of the low back pain and radiculopathy.

Currently, there are three modalities for imaging a herniated disc and disc fragments: myelography, computed tomography, and magnetic resonance imaging.

Our CT experience has been with the GE 8800 and the GE 9900; currently both our units are GE 9900. All our scans are made with angulation parallel to the intervertebral disc at each level; this is often impossible to attain at L5-S1. The 8800 scans were made using 5-mm thick slices every 4 mm, giving an overlap of 1 mm. The 9800 scans are 3 mm thick and are contiguous, without any overlap. Multimaging with soft tissue and bone windows are routine; reformatting is almost never employed.

Myelography is the oldest of these modalities and at one time was the only available method of diagnosis. It has several disadvantages. When a fragment is at the annulus level, the myelogram cannot distinguish it from an ordinary herniation. If the fragment is sequestered above or below the annulus, the myelogram may reveal a pressure deformity of the contrast column at a distance from the interspace (Figs. 3-2 and 3-3). This finding could be interpreted as a possible tumor or an inflammatory mass; a herniated fragment may be suspected if there is an appropriate clinical history.

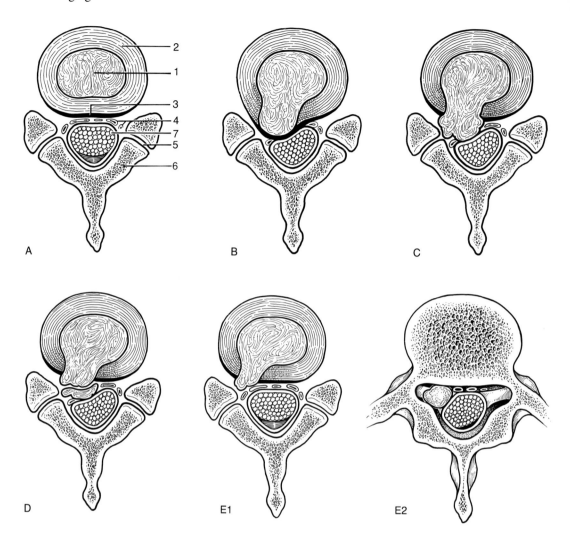

3-1 *(A)* Normal axial CT section. *(1)* Annular fibers. *(2)* Nucleus pulposis, *(3)* Posterior longitudinal ligament. *(4)* Epidural plexus. *(5)* Thecal sac (cauda equina). *(6)* Bony lamina. *(7)* Apophyseal joint.
(B) Simple herniated nucleus pulposis. The annular fibers are disrupted, but the posterior longitudinal ligament is intact although stretched.
(C) An extruded herniated nucleus pulposis. The herniation has perforated the posterior longitudinal ligament.

Often the posterior border of the herniation will appear irregular.
(D) An extruded fragment. A piece of the extrudend HNP has become detached, but is still lying at the level of the annulus.
(E) A sequestered fragment. (1) A small extruded herniation is seen at the level of the annulus. (2) About 1 cm below the annulus, a free fragment is lying against the right side of the thecal sac.

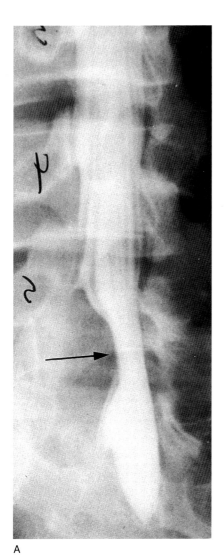

A

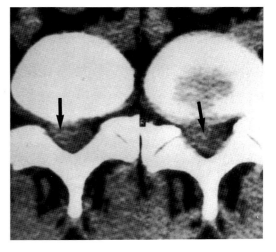

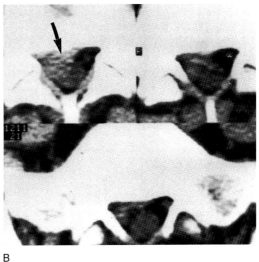

B

3-2 Fragment; myelographic appearance.
(A) The myelogram reveals indentation *(arrow)* of the right side of the contrast column most marked in the vicinity of the middle of L5. This defect is consistent with a mass lesion, including tumor, inflammatory mass, or a sequestered fragment from a herniated disc.

(B) On the CT scan the mass *(arrows)* has the appearance of a large disc fragment, which it proved to be on surgery.

37

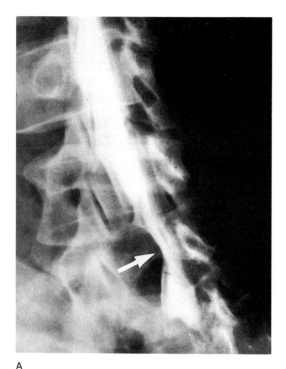

A

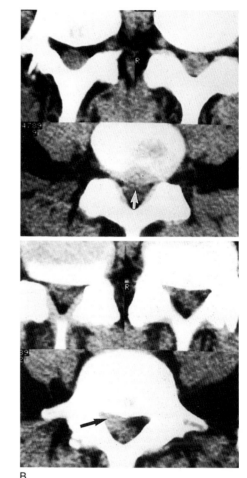

B

3-3 Myelogram of large disc fragment. This patient has a cauda equina syndrome. *(A)* Myelogram discloses large defect on the right side *(arrow)*. *(B)* CT at L4-L5 shows a central HNP *(white arrow)* and a large right-sided seques-tered fragment beginning about 9 mm below the annulus. *(C)* At L5-S1, the huge fragment *(arrows)* is seen extend-ing to just above the L5-S1 interspaace. Diagnosis from the myelogram alone would be uncertain.

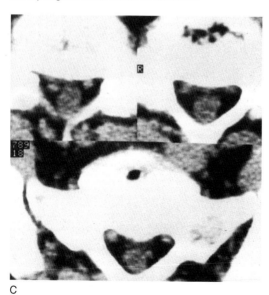

C

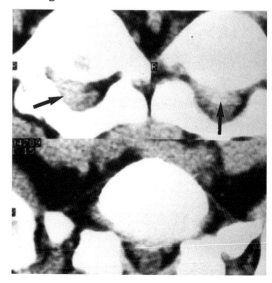

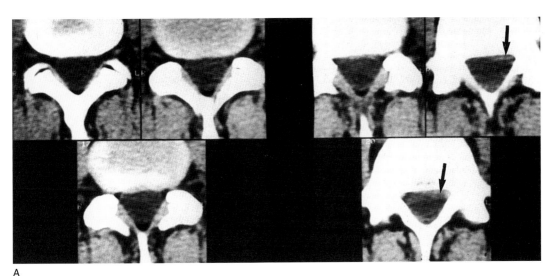

A

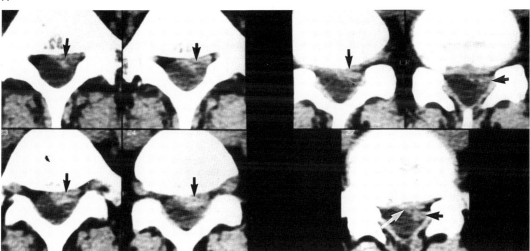

B

3-4 Huge fragment extending cephalad. *(A)* At L4-L5 the annulus is normal, but there is a left recess soft tissue density *(black arrows)* on the lowest two slices. *(B)* The L5-S1 scan shows a triangular density in the left anterior canal on all slices *(black arrows)*. On the last slice, just behind the herniation *(white arrow)* the bottom of the fragment *(black arrow)* is still visible. The fragment was at least 2.5 cm long!

If the sequestered fragment is not lying against the sac or pressing on a root, the myelogram will fail to disclose its presence.

Currently we believe that CT is the most reliable and accurate method for demonstrating a disc fragment (Fig. 3-4). However, with increasing experience, we have found that MRI can some-times clearly delineate a fragment at the annulus level when CT could not definitely disclose the fragmentation (Figs. 3-5 to 3-7).

The CT appearance of herniated disc fragments encompasses a wide spectrum. The fragment may be quite small and seen on only one slice; it may be huge, occasionally reaching a size of almost 2 cm.

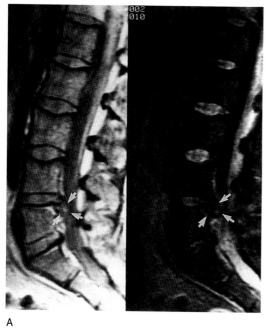

A

B

3-5 Extruded fragment on MRI. *(A)* The pair of sagittal slices (spin echo) left of midline clearly shows a large HNP fragment *(white arrows)* just caudad to the L4-L5 annulus.

(B) On the axial cuts, the fragment is clearly seen *(arrows)*.

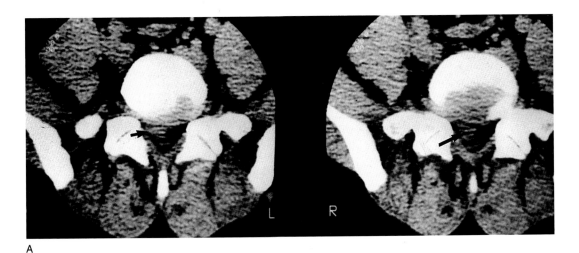

A

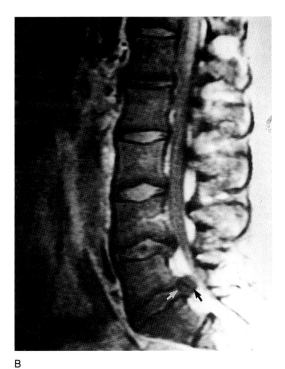

B

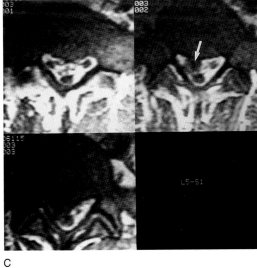

C

3-6　Extruded fragment, CT and MRI findings.
(A) At L5-S1, the CT reveals a right-sided herniation just touching the sac. It appears separated from the annulus.
(B) The sagittal MRI shows the herniation (black arrow)

separated from the annulus by a dark line (white arrow).
(C) The axial MR images at L5-S1 clearly show a round fragment (arrow) displacing the right S1 root posteriorly.

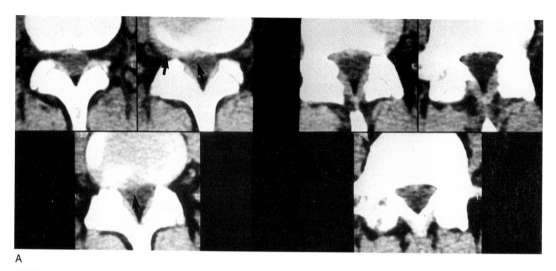

A

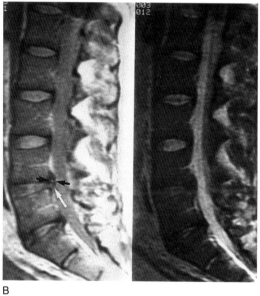

B

3-7 Fragment recognized on MRI but not on CT.
(A) The CT scans of L4-L5 show a central-right HNP *(black arrows).*
(B) The sagittal MRI clearly shows a small fragment *(black arrows)* above and contiguous to the protruded annulus *(white arrow).*

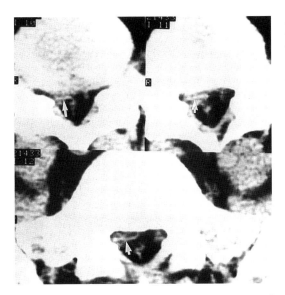

3-8 Linear fragment resembling a thickened epidural vessel. The density in the right anterior canal *(arrows)* of L5-S1 was a linear herniated disc fragment.

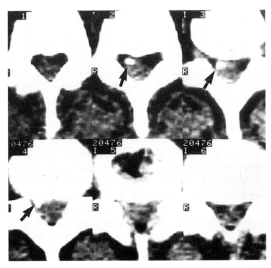

3-9 Calcified herniated disc fragment. The L3-L4 CT scan shows a calcification overlying the right anterior thecal sac on three slices *(arrows)*. No definite HNP was seen at the annulus level. At surgery, the calcifications proved to be calcified disc fragments. Such fragments are rare, since a calcified HNP is unlikely to fragment.

A fragment may be either well above or well below the annulus. Some of the larger fragments extend both above and below the annulus. When a fragment is contiguous to the annulus or to the herniation, it may be difficult or impossible to recognize it as a separate fragment (7); in this situation, the MRI may be more definitive (Fig. 3-7). If the anterior portion of the herniation is rounded or if a space is seen between it and the main herniation, identification of the fragment on CT is much easier. Although most fragments are soft tissue masses, occasionally the fragment may be entirely linear and may resemble a displaced epidural plexus (Fig. 3-8). A totally calcified fragment (Fig. 3-9) may be a puzzling finding but is extremely rare, since a calcified herniated nucleus polposus (HNP) is quite unlikely to break away from the annulus.

An interesting finding is a large rounded fragment which completely displaces and superficially resembles the thecal sac. This type of fragment will cause complete myelographic block. The fragment has a higher density than the thecal sac, which may allow identification of the fragment even when its shape and position strongly resemble the thecal sac. The increased density of the thecal sac (actually the fragment) could also be mistaken for an artefact. A repeat CT scan using thinner 1.5-mm slices or an MRI will usually clarify the issue. If still in doubt, a myelogram will reveal a complete block of the contrast at this level and will clarify the diagnosis (Fig. 3-10). However, this study is usually unnecessary if both CT and MRI studies are available.

One case was encountered in which the fragment apparently migrated from the right to the left side (Fig. 3-11).

When the disc fragment extends through the neural foramen, it may superficially resemble a conjoined root, a neurofibroma (Fig. 3-12), or an enlarged nerve root (Fig. 3-13) on the CT scan. However, a careful scrutiny of the annulus will usually reveal some irregularity or evidence of herniation. Sometimes a defect or asymmetrical irregularity in the annulus or herniation will suggest that a fragment has broken off. When no abnormality of the annulus or evidence of herniation can be seen and when the sequestered fragment is lying in the canal adjacent to the sac,

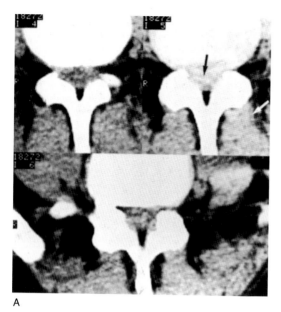

A

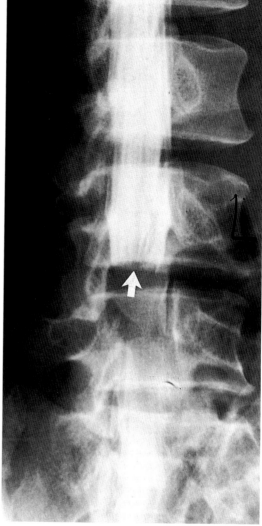

3-10   Extruded fragment simulating the thecal sac.
(A) Sequential CT slices of L3-L4 show a marked increase in the density of the "thecal sac" *(black arrow)* on one slice. Because of the somewhat increased density of the left paraspinal muscle *(white arrow),* the "sac" density was considered an artefact.
(B) Myelogram, performed because of severe clinical symptoms, shows a complete block at L3-L4. At surgery, a huge fragment had completely blocked the thecal sac. This fragment had been the dense "thecal sac."

B

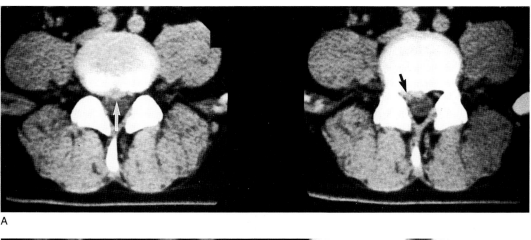

A

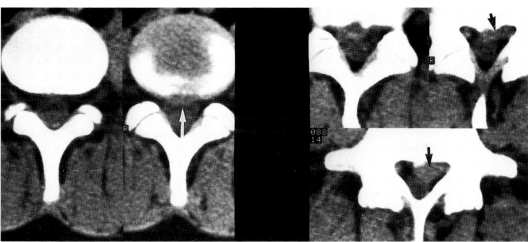

B

3-11 Migration of an extruded fragment.
(A) The L4-L5 scan shows a central HNP *(white arrow)* and a right-sided extruded fragment *(black arrow)*. There were right-sided symptoms.

(B) Three years later left-sided symptoms developed. The CT scan now shows the same central HNP *(white arrow),* but now there is a left-sided fragment *(black arrows)* but not right fragment. Presumably, the fragment migrated from the right to the left side of the canal!

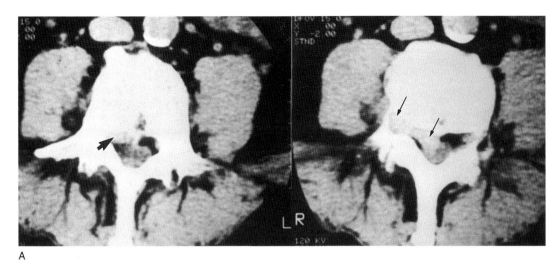

A

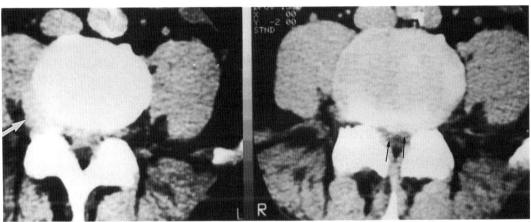

B

3-12 Fragment simulating a neurofibroma.
(A) A soft tissue mass in the right recess *(arrow)* is seen extending through the right neural foramen *(thin arrows)*. *(B)* The mass is extending into the paravertebral fat *(white arrow)*. Note the irregularity of the annulus *(thin arrows)*, which should have been a clue to the origin of the mass. A diagnosis of neurofibroma was entertained, but in keeping with the irregular annulus, the mass proved to be a sequestered fragment.

confident distinction from a tumor or inflammatory mass may be impossible. Clarification can usually be obtained by the use of intravenous enhancement CT. With proper enhancement technique virtually every neoplasm (benign or malignant) or inflammatory mass will enhance strongly, while a fragment, devoid of a blood supply, will not enhance. Strong enhancement occurs whenever tissue contains neovasculature which virtually always has much greater permeability than normal vasculature; consequently, in all neovascularized tissue, whether granulation, scar, tumor, or inflammatory tissue, the contrast material, if maintained at high levels in the circulation for several minutes, will pass through the permeable capillaries into the tissue substance and cause enhancement (6)!! Normal tissue and a herniated disc will at most enhance only slightly; a detached fragment will not enhance (Figs. 3-14 and 3-15).

What is the role of MRI in the detection of herniated disc fragments? With increasing experience, we find that MRI can sometimes distinguish

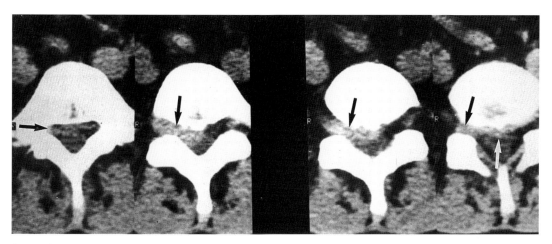

3-13 Fragment resembling an enlarged nerve root sleeve. The density in the right neural foramen *(black arrow)* of L5-S1 and extending about 9 mm above the annulus resembles an enlarged nerve root. However, its high density was more consistent with a herniated disc fragment, which it proved to be on surgery.

a fragment at the annulus level more covincingly than CT.

As mentioned above, occasionally a fragment lying contiguous to the main herniation cannot be distinguished as a separate fragment on the CT study. In such cases, on the sagittal sections of the MR a dark line (low signal) can be seen separating the fragment from the main herniation or from the nucleus pulposus (Fig. 3-7). A sequestered fragment should be recognized as easily on MRI as on CT (Fig. 3-6).

Our experience with fragments of a herniated disc can be summarzied as follows:

1. Recognition of an extruded fragment is important especially if percutaneous discectomy or chemonucleolysis is being considered. In the presence of a symptomatic fragment these procedures are ineffective.

2. Fragments are best demonstrated by high resolution CT studies. However, MRI may sometimes reveal fragmentation of a herniation when it cannot be clearly demonstrated on CT.

3. Myelography is much less useful than CT or MRI for confident evaluation of fragments. If a sequestered fragment is not pressing on the thecal sac it cannot be recognized. If the fragment is well above or below the annulus and presses on the sac, it may resemble a tumor or inflammatory mass on myelography. Fragmentation at the annulus level cannot be recognized on the myelogram.

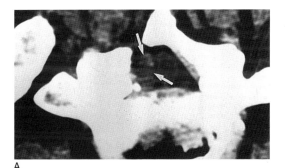

A

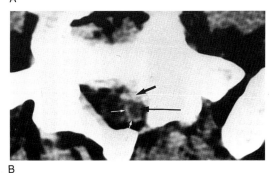

B

3-14 Postoperative mass in canal, intravenous enhancement. *(A)* CT of L5-S1 shows an oval soft tissue mass *(white arrows)* just left of the thecal sac. There has been a left laminectomy.

(B) CT after intravenous enhancement shows enhancing scar tissue in the left recess *(short black arrow)*. The epidural mass shows enhancement only of its medial border; the bulk of the mass *(long black arrow)* does not enhance, indicating that it is a herniated disc fragment and not a tumor.

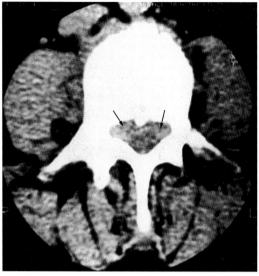

A

B

3-15   Tumor versus disc fragment, intravenous enhancement study. *(A)* The CT scan shows a soft tissue density *(arrows)* filling the anterior canal. The thecal sac is displaced posteriorly. The patient had a history of breast carcinoma, and it was unclear whether this anterior canal density was an HNP fragment or an epidural metastasis, even though no other metastases were found.

(B) Intravenous enhancement shows intense enhancement of the anterior canal density, confirming that it is an epidural metastasis. Radiation therapy relieved the symptoms; the epidural mass disappeared.

4. Occasionally a fragment may resemble an enlarged nerve root sleeve, conjoined root, a neurofibroma, or even an epidural tumor. If necessary, the latter two can be distinguished from a fragment by an intravenous enhanced CT study. Myelography or an MR study should help identify an enlarged nerve root sleeve.

References

1. Dillon, WP, Kaseff, LG et al.: Computed tomography and differential diagnosis of the extruded lumbar disc. *J. Comput Assist. Tomogr.* 7:969–975, 1983

2. Kambin, P, Sampson, S.: Posterolateral percutaneous suction-excision of herniated lumbar intervertebral discs. *Clin. Orthop.* 207:37–43, 1986.

3. Peyster, RO, Teplick, JG, Haskin, ME: Computed tomography of lumbosacral conjoined nerve root anomalies: Potential cause of false positive reading for herniated nucleus pulposis. *Spine* 10:331–337, 1985.

4. Teplick, JG, Haskin, ME: CT and lumbar disc herniation. *Radiol. Clin. North Am.* 21:259–388, 1983.

5. Teplick, JG, Haskin, ME: Computed tomography of the postoperative lumbar spine. *A.J.N.R.* 4:1053–1065, 1984.

6. Teplick, JG, Haskin, ME: Intravenous enhancement of the postoperative lumbar spine. *A.J.R.* 143:845–855, 1984.

7. Teplick, JG, Teplick, SK et al.: Pitfalls and unusual findings in computed tomography of the lumbar spine. *J. Comput. Assist. Tomogr.* 6:888–893, 1982.

4   CT/Discography of the Lumbar Spine

Richard D. Guyer

Despite being introduced over 50 years ago, discography, and more recently CT/discography, remains a controversial diagnostic modality. In more recent years, however, discography has become popular but still has clinicians divided as to its clinical significance. The controversy arises not so much from discography as a diagnostic modality, but from the standpoint of recommending a fusion based on an abnormal discogram in the face of other normal studies.

Historical Perspective

In 1948 discography was first described by Lindblom as a useful diagnostic modality to identify ruptures that could not be determined by myelography, especially at the L5-S1 level where there was a high incidence of false-negative myelograms (19). Subsequently, Wise and Weiford (35) in the United States published their experience with discography in 1951. It was further popularized by Collis and Gardner (4) who reported on their analysis of 1000 cases in 1962. Holt (14) in 1968, published his very controversial study, "The question of lumbar discography." His finding of a 37% false-positive rate of discography in asymptomatic volunteers has been used to discredit lumbar discography as a valid diagnostic study. There were, however, many methodological deficits in the study as elucidated later by Simmons et al. (27) in 1988. In 1970, Crock (6,7) described the "internal disc disruption syndrome," in which an annular tear could be diagnosed by discography. Thies was also discussed by Park et al. (23) in 1979. In 1971, Hartman et al. (13) had described the use of discography and found it useful in discovering unsuspected degenerated discs which were then included in primary fusion procedures, and was also useful in detecting clinically unsuspected disc protrusions. In 1975, Pat-

rick (24) reported on the use of discography being helpful in the detection of extreme lateral ruptures of lumbar herniated disc in which myelography was not helpful. Simmons and Segil (26) also in 1975 felt that discography was helpful in the localization of symptomatic levels of discogenic disease, the assessment of adjacent levels to contemplated fusion, determining painful pseudarthrosis, distinguishing organic versus psychological sources of pain, and defining the pain in scoliosis. Brodsky and Binder (2) in 1979 felt that lumbar discography provided important information when clinical symptoms existed, even in the face of negative myelography. Kostuik (18), in 1979 as well, reported that dicography was helpful in assessing complex pain problems and led to improved results of surgery in adult scoliotic patients due to more careful delineation of their problems.

Present State of the Art

In the 1980's papers began to appear in the literature combining both discography and axial computerized tomography. McCutcheon and Thompson (21), in 1985, felt that CT scanning was a useful adjunct in evaluating the lumbar spine. In 1987, Sachs, et al. (25,30) from the Texas Back Institute reported a clinical grading system for CT/discography. Since that time there have been numerous other articles published on this combined diagnostic technique. It delineates the internal pathology of the disc more clearly than routine AP and lateral films. Oftentimes small fissures within the annulus are not clearly detected by ordinary film radiography.

At the Texas Institute, we have investigated discography extensively. In 1988, we reported disc deterioration in low back syndromes, finding that in 56% of patients with nonspecific low back

49

pain and 59% of patients with low back and leg pain but without evidence of clinical radiculopathy were found to have both positive discographic pain provocation and moderate or severe disc deterioration. It was felt that intradiscal pathology played a significant role in such nonspecific low back pain syndromes (28). In another study, 107 low back patients were evaluated to determine whether or not disc narrowing correlated with degenerative disc disease. It was found that disc height did correlate significantly with degenerative annular changes, but disc height was a poor method for detecting early painful degenerative changes, that is, the early stages of degeneration were not manifested by disc space narrowing (32). In 1989 it was further reported that in a series of 291 patients, normal discs were usually painless, as was found in 86% of the cases. With increasing age, however, the proportion of severely degenerated discs that were painless increased. This would seem to explain the poor correlation of low back pain with radiographic degenerative changes reported in previous epidemiological studies (31). Also in 1989, the sensitivity and specificity of CT/discographic images were reported with the radiographic picture and the provoked pain studied. It was found that the sensitivity in detecting clinically painful discs was 89.6%, while the specificity was 62.3%. The latter figure was reflective, in part, of the number of discs producing dissimilar pain but having a positive image (12). In an additional study, the sensitivity and specificity of CT/discographic and myelographic images were compared on the basis of the pain provocation result. CT/discography showed an 87.6% sensitivity rate compared to 43% of all myelographic images. However, when comparing the specificity, CT/discography was only 55%, while myelography was 77.8% (29).

Walsh et al. (33) in 1989, reported a study determining the sensitivity and specificity of CT/discography. In this controlled prospective study of normal volunteers, as well as symptomatic patients, the false-positive rate of discography was determined. Results showed that 17% (5 of 30) of discs in the asymptomatic individuals and 50% of the total number of subjects (5 of 10) demonstrated abnormal images by CT/discography. In none of these patients however, was significant pain pro-

duced with the injection. Therefore, the false-positive rate was 0%, making the specificity 100%. In the symptomatic samples, 65% (13 of 20) of discs and 100% (7 of 7) of subjects demonstrated abnormal CT/discographic images at one or more levels. The false-positive rate, however, could not be determined. In this study the combination of self-reported pain and the rating of observed pain behaviors were both a reliable and valid evaluation procedure. In essence, the investigation repeated Holt's study, but with a carefully controlled and well-executed experimental protocol. They also noted that there was a high incidence of abnormal images in the asymptomatic population. However, when the pain response was considered in the evaluation of the discogram, the results were quite different. The study emphasized the importance of defining the patient's pain response during discography. In summary, the authors felt discography may be contraindicated for patients who had previous disc surgery at the level of injection, and finally, it showed that clinicians who "diagnose disc involvement solely on the basis of abnormal MR or CT evaluations will err in the diagnosis as much as 50% of the time" (33).

Calhoun et al. (3), in 1988, reported on the use of provocative discography in planning operations of the spine. For 137 patients in whom discography identified symptomatic disc disease, 121 (89%) had significant clinical benefit from surgery, while 16 did not. Of 25 patients in whom a technically successful operation had been performed on nonsymptomatic but morphologically abnormal discs, only 52% (11) had significant symptomatic relief, while 48% (G. Gibson, Personal communication, 1989) had no clinical benefit. Again this reinforces the fact that a positive discogram is one that (a) has abnormal morphology and (b) causes reproduction of the patient's symptoms.

Also in 1989 Bernard (1) reported a comparative study of CT scanning, myelography, CT/myelography, discography, and CT/discography in patients with ruptured discs. It was found that CT/discography was the most accurate test, being highly specific to an 89% level, but having low sensitivity of approximately 43%. It was suggested that CT/discography should be considered in patients with suspected disc herniation when other tests were nondiagnosive, especially those with a possible foraminal or recurrent herniated disc.

With the advent of MRI, it was felt that this would eliminate the need for discography. There have been several studies to date that show even in the presence of "normal MRI scan" a painful disc may still be detected by discography, i.e., a disc in which there is an annular tear. This has been reported by Zucherman et al. (36), in 1988, in which 18 patients were identified in whom MR scanning did not accurately reflect internal disc architecture or predict a response to the disc injection. All patients were found to have peripheral annular tears with or without small herniations and degenerative changes on the discogram or CT/discogram. Likewise, Bernard (1) in his paper also described 18 of 170 discs with normal image on MRI, but which were discographically abnormal, with CT/discography revealing annular tears or radial fissuring. Our experience at Texas Back Institute has been the same. (J Flemming, RD Guyer, et al.: MRI Versus CT/discography in assessing chronic lumbar pain, Unpublished data, 1989).

Current Perspectives

Why is there controversy? It appears that the present controversy of discography remains as it has in years past. If a patient was assumed to have an abnormal disc, then it was felt that this was his source of pain; therefore, it was believed that the patient would benefit from surgery and, in most cases, either anterior or posterior fusion. The diagnostic features of discography have been almost totally overlooked by those who equate abnormal discography with fusion. Those individuals, however, who have sought a more intellectual curiosity concerning discography have helped to promote interest in it as well as determining its usefulness. Surely the mechanism of pain production in the lumbar spine is far from clear. In 1988, Weinstein (34) reported in his study on the pain of discography that vasoactive intestinal peptide and substance P found in the dorsal root ganglion were affected indirectly by manipulations of the intervertebral disc and, therefore, that the pain of

abnormal discography may well be in part related to the chemical environment within the disc and the sensitized site of its nociceptors. It has been proven in many studies that a patient who has had exact pain reproduction at a disc level can undergo fusion and obtain a very acceptable result. We unfortunately are not talking about a 98% success rate as with total hip replacement but, nonetheless, a procedure which improves the quality of life for the individual. Regrettably, there are many mixed feelings conjured up as one contemplates fusions, especially when associated with workman's compensation injuries. Many authors, as well as our own group (20), have reported a greater than 70% success with type of surgery. Calhoun et al. (3) have reported an 88% success rate in those patients demonstrating positive discography. Collis and Gardner (5) reported a 90% result in fusing those patients with painful symptomatic degenerative discs.

Detractors of discography point to the lack of true randomized, double-blind, controlled studies. In fact, Nachemson (22) states that at the present time the only surgical procedures for the treatment of low back pain and sciatica that has been proven to be successful for relief of pain in a scientific manner, has been the excision of the herniated disc giving root pain. It is difficult to carry out such scientific studies in clinical situations when so many variables must be considered. Nonetheless, they are needed.

The other issue, however, that is not controversial is the use of discography as a diagnostic modality. This must be clearly separated from the assumed equation of discography and fusion. Discography is an excellent study for (a) determining lateral disc ruptures not seen by CT or myelography, (b) determining recurrent disc ruptures, especially when the diagnosis remains equivocal by other studies (c) determining symptomatic pseudarthrosis (16), and (d) clarifying any case where the routine diagnostic procedure, such as CT, MRI, and myelography, are not elucidative. Discography is also useful in (e) fusion to make certain that the integrity of the disc adjacent to the prospective fusion level is normal. Finally, discography is helpful in (f) determining whether or not a disc is contained or extruded, which in the past was helpful in determining the appropriateness of chemonucleolysis and more recently whether a patient is a candidate for percutaneous discectomy.

To date, CT/discography is the only study that allows true anatomy of the disc to be determined. It can diagnose early annular tears that cannot be determined even on present MRI scans. It stands to reason that if some individuals are experiencing back pain, the only signs of degeneration could be an early annular tear, which is the beginning of the degenerative cascade as discussed by Kirkaldy-Willis et al. (17). This does not, however, dictate the type of treatment that would be best for the patient. This is where scientific studies are needed. Just as ligamentous injuries can repair and remodel with rehabilitation, it is not unreasonable to assume that annular tears may well respond to the same type of treatment. With the advent of functional rehabilitation, this may be the answer for such early injuries.

Safety of Discography

There have been some concerns about the incidence of infection, and in a study I reported in 1988, there is an incidence of 0.1%. This has been achieved only through the use of the same team of radiologists and strict aseptic techniques (11).

There have been excellent animal experimental studies carried out by Fraser et al. (8,9). First in 1987, and with a follow-up in 1989, they reported at the International Society for the Study of Lumbar Spine that discitis is a result of bacterial contamination. They suggested a single dose of cephlosporin was indicated at the time of discography, administered either intradiscally or intravenously. In their hands the incidence of infection was slightly greater than 3% and was reduced several fold with the use of antibiotics. Our personal experience was that the incidences were so low that antibiotics are not recommended in lumbar discography (11).

It also has been questioned whether or not discography can injure the disc. In an experimental dog study by Garrick and Sullivan (10) in 1970, it was shown that there was no evidence of microscopic degenration one year after discography. In another study, with the follow-up of patients who

had undergone previous discography, Johnson (15) reported in 1988 that in 42 repeat discograms, only one was found to be truly abnormal in the second study. The author concluded that there is no evidence that diagnostic discography damaged a normal disc.

Finally, as Nachemson (22) pointed out, there is the concern over radiation exposure for such a diagnostic study. To date, there is no correlation between multiple diagnostic studies, whether they be spine-related or other radiographic examinations, in the development of disease later in life (G Gibson, Personal communication, 1989).

Usefulness in Percutaneous Discectomy

As is discussed in other chapters of this book, percutaneous discectomy is best performed in those patients who have a contained disc rupture, that is, a disc in which the nucleus is still sealed within the confines of the annulus. CT scanning is not always helpful in determining whether or not the disc is extruded or contained. Even with high-quality, thin cut CT scanning, it still stretches the limits of the clinician's acuity to be 100% certain that the disc is contained. With present day MR scanning this is becoming less of a problem, although there are still those equivocal cases for which the diagnosis cannot be easily made. If all clinicians had access to excellent quality MR scans and CT scans, the diagnosis might be more easily found, but this is not the reality.

The following examples illustrate some of the diagnostic dilemmas that the clinician faces and how CT/discography can aid in the diagnosis and decision-making process.

Case 1

The first is a 30-year-old patient, P. H., who had primarily right leg pain. He was initially evaluated using CT scanning which showed a central protrusion, but the extent of it was difficult to determine (Fig. 4-1). He therefore underwent CT/discography which showed leakage of the dye about a large central disc herniation (Fig. 4-2); therefore, the patient was not felt to be a candidate for percutane-

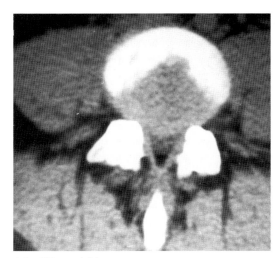

4-1 CT scan L4-L5.

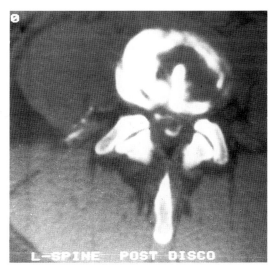

4-2 CT discogram showing dye extravasating about extruded fragment L4-L5.

ous discectomy, and at surgery a large extruded disc fragment was identified.

Case 2

In the next case, a 41-year-old patient complained of right buttock and right thigh aching. Her MR scan showed a central protrusion at L5-S1. She

had a normal EMG and nerve conduction study and, therefore, underwent myelography with follow-up CT scanning that showed a moderate central disc protrusion at L5-S1. Feeling that there was still not enough information to offer the patient any kind of intervention, she underwent CT/discography that reproduced her buttock and leg pain (Fig. 4-3). She was, therefore, felt to be a candidate for percutaneous discectomy which proved to provide complete resolution of her leg symptoms.

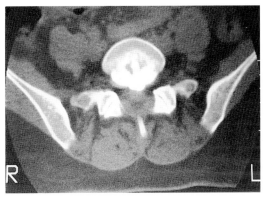

4-3 CT discogram showing central rupture L5-S1.

Case 3

Finally, the next patient is a 56-year-old patient who complained of severe left buttock and right calf pain. During hospitalization, the etiology of his pain was unclear. He was noted to have diminished pulses in the right leg and was evaluated by the vascular service, which concluded that he had atherosclerotic partial occlusion of the right iliac. Because of the severity of his pain with weight bearing, he underwent a lumbar CT (Fig. 4-4) that was suggestive of a small lateral disc herniation. Myelography was carried out that was unremarkable. The patient failed to improve with further conservative treatment, but the diagnosis was still unclear. He then underwent CT/discography and had pain reproduction of his hip and leg pain. The protrusion was clearly seen on the discogram (Fig. 4-5). He subsequently underwent an open discectomy, but, in retrospect, had

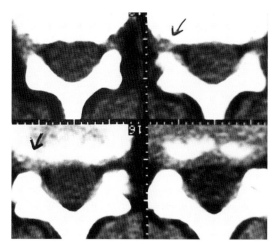

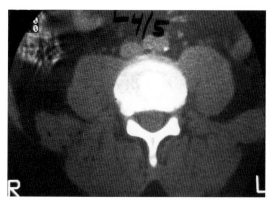

4-5 CT discogram L4-L5 confirming lateral disc rupture.

4-4 CT scan L4-L5 showing probable lateral disc rupture right L4-L5.

percutaneous discectomy been available, I feel the patient may have been a candidate for such.

Summary

CT/discography as it is now carried out is a sophisticated study that allows the clinician to determine the internal structure of the disc as no other study to date can allow. One can clearly define early degenerative disc disease before plain x-rays would show any abnormalities. It is useful for those patients who have recurrent discs, who have had previous surgery, or who have unexplained symptoms despite multiple other diagnostic studies. It can clarify equivocal lateral disc ruptures and identify symptomatic pseudarthroses. It is also a useful adjunct for those patients in whom a fusion is contemplated, making certain that the fusion is carried to a normal level and not an abnormal level, and also in determining whether or not a disc is contained and therefore whether or not the patient is a candidate for percutaneous discectomy.

It remains an excellent diagnostic modality when coupled with the determination of the patient's pain reproduction. In essence, it is analogous to early arthroscopy in which one saw the early degenerative changes of the knee joint but yet the plain x-rays and arthrograms were negative. These patients complained of pain, and it was felt that their complaints did correlate with the early degenerative abnormalities seen. Herein lies the analogy to discography. The controversial part, however, has been heated in the past concerning the equation of discography with surgical fusion. While these patients cannot be "cured of their pain" a substantial number of them can be helped. It is difficult to carry out true controlled prospective randomized clinical trials when one is dealing with subjective complaints such as pain, along with a myriad of other variables, but this goal must be continually pursued.

References

1. Bernard, TN, Jr: Lumbar Discography and Post-discography Computerized Tomography: Refining the Diagnosis in Low Back Pain. Presented at the North American Spine Society, Quebec, Canada, June 1989.
2. Brodsky, AD, Binder, WF: Lumbar discography: Its value in diagnosis and treatment of lumbar disc lesions. *Spine* 4:110–120, 1979.
3. Calhoun, E, McCall, IW, Williams, L, Pullicino VN: Provocation discography as a guide to planning operations on the spine. *J. Bone Joint Surg.* 70B:267–271, 1988.
4. Collis, JS, Gardner, WJ: Lumbar discography. *JAMA* 178(1):67–69, 1961.
5. Collis, JS Jr, Gardner, WJ: Lumbar discography: An analysis of thousand cases. *J. Neurosurg.* 19:452, 1962.
6. Crock, HV: A reappraisal of intervetebral disc lesions. *Med. J. Aust.* 1:983–990, 1970.
7. Crock, HV: Internal disc disruption: A challenge to disc prolapse fifty years on. *Spine* 11(6):650–653, 1986.
8. Fraser, RD, Osti, OL, Vernon-Roberts, B: Discitis after discography. *J. Bone Joint Surg.* 69B:31–35, 1987.
9. Fraser, RD, Osti, OL, Vernon-Roberts, B: Iatrogenic Discitis – the Role of Intravenous Antibiotics in Prevention and Treatment: An Experimental Study. Presented at the International Society for the Study of the Lumbar Spine, Kyoto, Japan, May 1989.
10. Garrick, JG, Sullivan, CR: Long-term effects of diskography in dogs. *Minnesota Med* Aug:849–850, 1970.
11. Guyer, RD, Collier, R, Stith, WJ, Ohnmeiss, DD, Hochschuler, SG, Rashbaum, RF, Regan JJ: Discitis after discography. *Spine* 13(12):1352–1354, 1988.
12. Guyer, RD, Vanharanta, H, Ohnmeiss, DD, et al.: Sensitivity and Specificity of CT/Discography. Poster presentation at the North American Spine Society Conference, Quebec, Canada, June 1989.
13. Hartmann, JT, Kendrick, JI, Lorman, P: Discography as an aid in evaluation for lumbar and lumbosacral fusion. *Clin. Orthop.* 81:77–81, 1971.
14. Holt, EP Jr: The question of lumbar discography. *J. Bone Joint Surg.* 50A:720–726, 1968.
15. Johnson, RG: Does discography injure normal discs? An analysis of repeat discograms. *Spine* 14(4):424–426, 1989.
16. Johnson, RG, Macnab, I: Localization of symptomatic lumbar pseudarthrosis by use of discography. *Clin, Orthop.* 187:164–170, 1985.
17. Kirkaldy-Willis, WH, Paine, KWE, Cauchiox, J, McIvor, GWD: Lumbar spinal stenosis. *Clin. Orthop.* 99:30, 1974.
18. Kostuik, JP: Decision making in adult scoliosis. *Spine* 4(6):521–525, 1979.
19. Lindblom, K: Diagnostic puncture of intervertebral disks in sciatica. *Acta Orthop. Scand.* 17:231–239, 1948.
20. Loguidice, VA, Johnson, RG, Guyer, RD, Stith, WJ, Ohnmeiss, DD, Hochschuler, SH, Rashbaum, RF: Anterior lumbar interbody fusion. *Spine* 13(3):366–369, 1988.
21. McCutcheon, ME, Thomson, WC: CT scanning of lumbar discography: A useful diagnostic adjunct. *Spine* 11(3):257–259, 1986.
22. Nachemson, A: Editorial comment: Lumbar discography – Where are we today? *Spine* 14(6):555–557, 1989.
23. Park, WM, McCall, W, O'Brien, JP, Webb, JK: Fissuring of the posterior annulus fibrosis in the lumbar spine. *Br. J. Radiol.* 52:382–387, 1979.
24. Patrick, BS: Extreme lateral ruptures of lumbar intervertebral discs. *Surg. Neurol.* 3:301–304, 1975.
25. Sachs, B, Vanharanta, H, Spivey, M, et al.: Dallas Discogram Description: A new classification of CT/discography in low back disorders. *Spine* 12:287–294, 1987.
26. Simmons, EG, Segil, CM: An evaluation of discography in the localization of symptomatic levels in discogenic disease of the spine. *Clin. Orthop.* 108:57–69, 1975.
27. Simmons, JW, Aprill, CN, Dwyer, AP, Brodsky, AE: A reassessment of Holt's data on: "the question of lumbar discography." *Clin. Orthop.* 237:120, 1988.
28. Vanharanta, H, Guyer, RD, Ohnmeiss, DD, et al.: Disc deterioration in low-back syndromes: A prospective multi-center CT/discography study. *Spine* 13 (12): 1349–1351, 1988.
29. Vanharanta, H, Guyer, RD, Ohnmeiss, DD, Hochschuler, SH, Rashbaum, RF: Validity of myelographic and CT/discographic images in identifying clinically painful disc lesions. Submitted to *Spine* for publication, 1989.
30. Vanharanta, H, Sachs, B, Spivey, M, et al.: The relationship of pain provocation to lumbar disc deterioration as seen by CT/discogram. *Spine* 12:295–298, 1987.
31. Vanharanta, H, Sachs, BL, Ohnmeiss, DD, et al.: Pain provocation and disc deterioration by age: A CT/discography study in low-back pain population. *Spine* 14(4):420–423, 1989.

32. Vanharanta, H, Sachs, BL, Spivey, M, et al.: A comparison of CT/discography, pain response and radiographic disc height. *Spine* 13:321–324, 1988.

33. Walsh, TR, Weinstein, JN, Spratt, KF, et al.: Lumbar discography: A controlled, prospective study of normal volunteers to determine the false-positive rate. *Spine* in press, 1989.

34. Weinstein, J, Claverie, W, Gibson, S: The pain of discography. *Spine* 13:12, 1344–1348, 1988.

35. Wise, RE, Weiford, EC: X-ray visualization of the intervertebral disc: report of a case. *Cleve. Clin. Q.* 18:127, 1951.

36. Zucherman, J, Derby, R, Hsu, D, Picetti, G, Kaiser, J, Schofferman, J, Goldthwaite, N, White, A: Normal magnetic resonance imaging with abnormal discography. *Spine* 13(12):1355–1359, 1988.

SECTION III
ANESTHESIA

5 Choice of Anesthetics and Role of the Anesthesiologist in Percutaneous Lumbar Discectomy

John J. BianRosa and *John G. Goode*

There are over 20 million anesthetics performed in the United States each year; 2,000 of these patients die as a direct result of anesthesia complications. In fact, most Western nations experience nearly the same mortality rate of approximately one death per 10,000 cases (0.01%) (9). The majority of these deaths are the result of a combination of both technology-related and human error; a few are unavoidable because of patient disease, idiosyncrasy, or other as yet unexplained factors (12).

Various studies have revealed that between 50 to 82% of anesthetic deaths are due to preventable human error (4). A December 1985 review of anesthesia malpractice claims by the Pennsylvania Hospital Insurance Company (PHICO) found that human error appeared to be the most common cause of anesthesia-related death. A more recent study (1988) of closed claims involving major insurance losses by the American Society of Anesthesiologists (ASA) Committee on Professional Liability found that airway management represented the most common etiological factor in brain damage and death, and that better monitoring would have prevented at least 29% of the mishaps. It has become clear that, "the most common problem leading to anesthesia related injury, by far, is failure of adequate ventilation, whether from an unrecognized esophageal intubation, a breathing system disconnection, kinked or dislodged endotracheal tube or breathing system tubing, incorrect ventilator settings, or simply inadequate spontaneous or assisted ventilation under anesthesia" (7).

With the recognition of human and/or technical error in the etiology of anesthesia mishaps, an even greater emphasis is now being placed on anesthetist vigilance, which is the absolute foundation of anesthesia care, and the augmentation of this vigilant capacity through various ancillary monitoring aids. "While it is recognized that

monitoring with devices in no way replaces vigilance, any anesthesiologist can make a mistake that may be detected by an alarm before harm occurs" (15).

In 1985, in an attempt to improve patient safety and risk management, the Department of Anesthesia of Harvard Medical School adopted specific mandatory standards for minimal patient monitoring during anesthesia for all nine component teaching hospitals. The core of the Harvard standards is the emphasis on continuous monitoring of ventilation and circulation rather than intermittent observation (8). In the following year, 1986, the Federal Drug Administration (FDA) issued a Pre-Anesthesia Apparatus Checkout Procedure in the hope of reducing deaths and injuries attributable to preexisting equipment faults or to errors in equipment setup. The preanesthesia checkout procedure is only a recommendation and not a federal regulation, but common sense and prudence dictate its usage. By October 1986, the time had come for the American Society of Anesthesiologists to set National Standards for Basic Intraoperative Monitoring. Specific standards for continual evaluation of oxygenation, ventilation, circulation, and temperature of the patient during general, regional, and monitored anesthesia care were defined. Sedative or monitored anesthesia care (MAC) techniques require the same standards of care as general anesthesia. However, pulse oximetry and end-tidal CO_2 monitoring (capnography) are not required but only encouraged, a reflection of the fact that some hospitals may not be financially capable of securing them. The use of additional monitoring (pulse oximetry/capnography) may actually be cost-effective if patient injuries are reduced and savings in insurance costs are realized (19). Fortunately, anesthesia-related morbidity and mortality have begun to decline in the past several years because of recognition and better understanding of

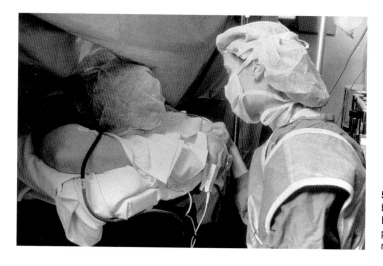

5-1 The following monitors have been applied to this patient: BP cuff, EKG leads, and pulse oximeter probe (left index finger), as well as nasal oxygen cannulae.

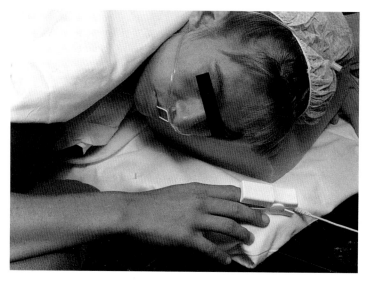

5-2 Oxygen cannulae with oral and nasal CO_2 sampling ports.

the risk of anesthesia and the efforts made to improve clinical behavior through education in patient safety and by development of new technology (15).

Percutaneous lumbar discectomy necessitates an anesthetic technique consisting of local anesthesia with conscious sedation, commonly referred to as monitored anesthesia care (MAC) (Fig. 5-1). The objective of conscious sedation is to produce a comfortable, cooperative amnestic patient who has an elevated pain threshold but who is still conscious and able to protect his or her air-

way. Intravenous conscious sedation is based on the principle of pharmacological titration whereby the least amount of drug necessary to reach the desired endpoint (sedation) is used.

Monitoring, as previously discussed, is necessary to ensure only minor variations in vital signs so that morbidity and mortality are avoided. As recommended by the ASA Standards of Monitoring (October 1986) we utilize the following monitors on a routine basis: *(a)* inspired gas oxygen analyzer; *(b)* continuous electrocardiogram; and *(c)* blood pressure (at least every five minutes). We also use end-tidal CO_2 and pulse oximetry monitors which are strongly encouraged by the ASA standards (Fig. 5-2).

CO_2 analyzers use the absorption of infrared light to measure CO_2, the amount of absorption being proportional to the CO_2 concentration (11). Ventilatory depression can be quantified, and apnea can be detected. Nasal O_2 cannulae can be modified by addition of either an intravenous catheter (10) or a syringe tip cap (1) to provide a sampling port. Data obtained with the latter setup provide CO_2 measurements which correlate with values obtained from arterial blood gas measurements. Salter labs (Arvin, CA) manufactures an oxygen nasal cannula (#4003) with built-in oral and nasal CO_2 sampling ports (Fig. 5-3).

The pulse oximeter combines oximetry (the spectrophotometric determination of hemoglobin saturation) with plethysmography (recording changes in tissue volume) to achieve virtually real-time measurements and display of two important physiological variables: heart rate and arterial oxygen saturation (11). "The oxygen saturation determination is based on the different spectrophotometric properties of oxyhemoglobin and reduced hemoglobin at a red (660 nm) and an infrared wavelength (920 nm)" (11). The instrument works by detecting the fluctuation in tissue volume associated with each pulse and the change in light transmitted from arterial blood (11). Analysis of light transmitted at both wavelengths leads to determination of arterial oxygen saturation. The probe may be attached to any pulsatile tissue, including finger, toe, nose, or ear. Saturation and PO_2 are related according to the oxyhemoglobin dissociation curve.

The local anesthetic which is most commonly used is 1% lidocaine with epinephrine. Approximately 10 cc are required. This local anesthetic is used to anesthetize the skin and muscle layers along the path of introduction of surgical instruments. Onset of anesthesia is rapid, and duration of anesthesia is approximately 75 minutes. The upper limit for safe dosage in the adult is 200 to 400 mg (20). The total dose of lidocaine should not exceed 6.4 mg/kg which is the threshold dose producing CNS symptoms in humans (17). Toxic symptoms such as visual disturbances and muscular twitching occur at blood concentrations above

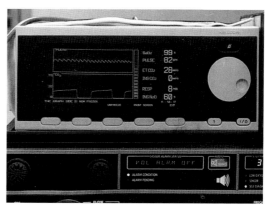

5-3 Nellcor multi-function monitor which measures oxygen saturation, pulse rate, end tidal CO_2 level, and respiratory rate. The top left graph represents plethmysography data (changes in tissue volume) whereas the lower left graph represents end tidal CO_2 levels.

5 µg/ml, and convulsions occur at concentrations greater than 10 µg/ml (20). Lidocaine is metabolized in the liver.

For conscious sedation, a combination of fentanyl and midazolam is utilized. Fentanyl provides analgesia during infiltration with lidocaine as well as during surgery. Midazolam reduces anxiety and provides amnesia.

Fentanyl is a synthetic opiod related to the phenylpiperidines (21). Fentanyl is 80 times as potent as morphine and 1000 times as potent as meperidine (21). Because fentanyl is highly lipid-soluble, it enters the nervous system rapidly and has an almost immediate onset of action when administered intravenously (13). Although doses from 1 to 10 µg/kg of fentanyl produce analgesia, doses as large as 30 to 100 µg/kg have been used with oxygen and pancuronium (a muscle relaxant) as a total anesthetic for cardiac surgery. After a single intravenous dose of 100 µg, the analgesic effect usually lasts from 30 to 60 minutes. Side effects of fentanyl include respiratory depression, bradycardia secondary to stimulation of the central vagal nucleus in the medulla, emesis due to stimulation of the chemoreceptor trigger zone (less than 4%), and chest wall rigidity (usually dose-dependent) (2,13). The respiratory system demonstrates a dose-dependent decrease in responsiveness of the brainstem respiratory center to carbon dioxide. The peak respiratory depressant effect occurs from

5 to 15 minutes following IV-injection, but respiratory depression persists longer than the analgesic effect (13). Although fentanyl, morphine, and meperidine produce approximately the same degree of respiratory depression at equianalgesic doses, fentanyl produces much less cardiovascular depression. Virtually all hemodynamic variables remain stable during fentanyl administration (cardiac output, blood pressure, and filling pressures) (13). Fentanyl, unlike morphine, has no effect on histamine release.

An overdose of fentanyl can be treated with naloxone (Narcan), a pure antagonist which competes for the same receptor sites (14). By titrating with small doses, reversal of respiratory depression can be obtained with the preservation of analgesia and avoidance of unpleasant symptoms, such as nausea, vomiting, and extreme hypertension.

Fentanyl is metabolized in the liver and is excreted in the urine primarily as metabolites and, to a lesser extent, as the unchanged drug (13).

"Midazolam (Versed) is a short acting water soluble benzodiazepine and a member of a new class of imidazobenzodiazepine derivatives" (6). This drug, which is approximately 2 to 3 times as potent as diazepam, was synthesized in 1976 by Fryer and Walser but was not marketed until 1986. "At a pH below four, part of the drug in solution has an open benzepine ring thus imparting water solubility, but at physiologic pH the whole of the drug is present in closed-ring form and the lipid solubility of the drug is increased" (6). Thus, this drug, unlike diazepam, does not have to be prepared in propylene glycol and is not painful on IV injection. "The high lipophilicity of midazolam at physiological pH causes it to have a very rapid onset of activity after IV administration. In experimental models, the drug rapidly enters the cerebral spinal fluid and equilibration between plasma and CSF generally occurs within a few minutes of IV administration. Midazolam's entry into brain tissue and the onset of clinical effects are correspondingly rapid" (16). The average dose required for intravenous sedation is 0.05 mg/kg, whereas doses of 0.15 to 0.4 mg/kg have been used for induction of general anesthesia. Side effects include respiratory depression, apnea (related to dose and speed of injection), and hemodynamic

changes including decreased systemic vascular resistance and a reflex increase in heart rate. There is evidence from volunteers that low sedative doses of midazolam used alone, 0.075 mg/kg IV, do not affect the ventilatory response to CO_2 (16).

The ability to produce a short period of anterograde amnesia is a useful feature of both midazolam and diazepam when used for sedation. Patients have little or no memory of the unpleasant injection of local anesthesia or passage of surgical instruments (6). Numerous studies have shown that midazolam has a more rapid onset of sedation and a much greater degree of amnesia than diazepam (3,5,6).

An overdose of midazolam may be treated with a specific antagonist, RO 15–1788 (not commercially available yet), or with physostigmine (Antilirium). Physostigmine antagonizes midazolam nonspecifically via a cholinergic mechanism (i.e., inhibition of acetylcholinesterase) (16).

Midazolam metabolism involves both hydroxylation and glucuronidation in the liver (16). These metabolites are excreted in the urine with very little intact drug excreted unchanged. The plasma half-life of midazolam is two to five hours, whereas the plasma half-life of diazepam is 20 to 99 hours (6).

There is no empirical formula for administration of midazolam and fentanyl during anesthesia for percutaneous lumbar discectomy. We routinely administer nasal oxygen, since our experience as well as one clinical study have shown significant drops in arterial oxygenation during sedation using the above two drugs (18). End-tidal CO_2 is also measured, since we expect some respiratory depression. A titration of drug vs. level of anxiety, degree of responsiveness, respiratory rate, oxygen saturation, end-tidal CO_2, and vital signs is carried out. Factors such as age (less drug with increasing age) and preexisting disease [midazolam may cause more prolonged respiratory depression in patients with chronic obstructive pulmonary disease (COPD)] (6) are taken into account. We plan to have a patient who is sedated (closed eyelids, unresponsive to light stimulation) and possibly dysarthric but still responsive and cooperative when necessary. Care must be taken to avoid oversedation which might lead to marked respiratory depression and inability to cooperate.

We tend to give most of our pharmacological therapy before infiltration with local anesthesia so that peaks in drug concentrations will be earlier. Thus, by the end of a procedure the concentrations and side effects of midazolam and fentanyl should be considerably reduced.

The range of drug administration is as follows:

fentanyl	1–5 µg/kg
midazolam	0.01–0.1 mg/kg

However, lower of higher doses may be indicated and arrived at by careful titration as stated above.

Some patients may require additional local anesthesia instead of sedation during surgery. This possibility should be thought of early before an overdose of sedatives is given.

We have found that the combination of local anesthesia (lidocaine) with powerful short-acting intravenous agents (fentanyl and midazolam) provides excellent conditions for surgery with minor side effects or complications when properly administered with appropriate monitoring and adherence to published ASA standards of care.

References

1. Blue, EA, Boysen, PG, Broome, JA, Klein, EF: Measurement of End Tidal CO_2 Using Modified Cannulae. New York State Society of Anesthesiology Annual Meeting, New York, 1987.
2. Campbell, R: Prevention of complications associated with intravenous sedation and general anesthesia. *J. Oral Maxillofac. Surg.* 44:289–301, 1986.
3. Clark, RN, et al.: A comparative study of intravenous diazepam and midazolam for oral surgery. *J. Oral Maxillofac. Surg.* 44:860–863, 1986.
4. Cooper, JB, Newbower, RS, Long, CD, et al.: Preventable anesthesia mishaps: A study of human factors. *Anesthesiology* 49:399–406, 1978.
5. Dixon, J, et al.: Sedation for local anesthesia. Comparison of intravenous midazolam and diazepam. *Anaesthesia* 39:372–376, 1984.
6. Dundee, JW, et al.: Midazolam, A review of its pharmacological properties and therapeutic use. *Drugs* 28:519–543, 1984.
7. Eichhorn, JH: Monitoring standards for clinical practice. *IARS* Review Course Lectures: 113–119, 1988.
8. Eichhorn, JH, Cooper JB, Cullen DJ, et al.: Standards for patient monitoring during anesthesia at Harvard Medical School. *JAMA* 256:1017–1020, 1986.
9. Emergency Care Research Institute: Death during general anesthesia. *J. Health Care Technol.* 1:155–175, 1985.
10. Goldman, JA: A simple, easy, and inexpensive method for monitoring $ETCO_2$ through nasal cannulae (letter). *Anesthesiology* 67:606, 1987.
11. Gravenstein, N: Gas. *In* Gravenstein, N (ed): *Problems in Anesthesia,* pp 47–59. JB Lippincott, Philadelphia, 1987.
12. Keats, AS: Role of anesthesia in surgical mortality. *In* Orkin, FK, Cooperman, LH (eds.): *Complications in Anesthesiology,* p 3. JB Lippincott, Philadelphia, 1983.
13. Miller, DL, Wall, RT: Fentanyl and diazepam for analgesia and sedation during radiologic special procedures. *Radiology* 162:195–198, 1987.
14. Moldenhauer, CC: New narcotic. *In* Kaplan, J (ed.): *Cardiac Anesthesia* p 69. Grune & Stratton, New York, 1983.
15. Pierce, ED: Risk modification in anesthesia. *Practice Management in Anesthesiology,* November 1987.
16. Reves, JG, Fragen, RJ, et al.: Midazolam: pharmacology and uses. *Anesthesiology* 62:310–324, 1985.
17. Savarese, JJ, Covino, B: Basic and clinical pharmacology of local anesthetic drugs. *In* Miller R (ed.): *Anesthesia,* (ed. 2, pp 984–1013. Churchill Livingstone, New York, 1986.
18. Tucker, MR, Ochs, MW, et al.: Arterial blood gas levels after midazolam or diazepam administered with or without fentanyl as an intravenous sedative for outpatient surgical procedures. *J. Oral Maxillofac. Surg.* 44:688–692, 1986.
19. Whitcher, C, Ream, AK, Parsons, D, et al.: Anesthesia mishaps and the cost of monitoring: A proposed standard for monitoring equipment. *J. Clin. Monit.* 4:5–15, 1988.
20. Wood, M: Local anesthetic agents. *In* Wood, M, Wood, A (eds.): *Drugs and Anesthesia,* pp 342–371. Williams & Wilkins, Baltimore, 1982.
21. Wood, M: Narcotic analgesics and antagonists. *In* Wood, M, Wood, A (eds.): *Drugs and Anesthesia,* p 184. Williams & Wilkins, Baltimore, 1982.

SECTION IV

Percutaneous Lumbar Discectomy

6 Posterolateral Percutaneous Lumbar Discectomy and Decompression: Arthroscopic Microdiscectomy

Parviz Kambin

Introduction

The percutaneous approach to the lumbar intervertebral discs is emerging as an acceptable method of treatment for symptom-producing herniated lumbar discs. In contrast to discectomy following laminectomy (31) and microlumbar discectomy (27) the spinal canal is not entered during the course of percutaneous discectomy. For this particular reason the posterolateral percutaneous approach has gained broad appeal.

Currently three basic instruments are available for percutaneous lumbar discectomy (PLD). In this chapter our experience and the detail of the operative technique will be discussed. This will be followed by two other approaches, namely biportal technique and the use of a straight automated nucleotome.

Although we have experience with and have utilized small caliber instruments in the early stages of our clinical work (4, 21), we have learned that the larger caliber working sheaths can be inserted into the intervertebral disc with relative safety. At this state of the art the larger working sheath appears to be necessary for accommodation of the instruments which are needed to reach posteriorly and posterolaterally for the evacuation of the offending fragments.

Percutaneous lumbar discectomy offers a new concept and technique in the armamentarium used for the treatment of herniated lumbar disc and its associated radiculopathy. However, lumbar laminectomy continues to be the cornerstone of treatment for sequestrated, extruded discs and spinal stenosis. (21, 23, 25).

The dynamic technical evolution both in the area of instrumentation and visualization has opened a new horizon in the field of percutaneous lumbar discectomy. The ongoing efforts and clinical research on this subject will undoubtedly bring about further scientific and technical refinement to this operative procedure.

Preoperative Care and Patient Selection

When surgical management of a symptom-producing herniated disc becomes necessary, the physician has the responsibility to educate the patient on the various surgical modalities which are currently available, namely, lumbar laminectomy, microlumbar discectomy, percutaneous lumbar discectomy, and chemonucleolysis.

Although in certain European Centers (32, 33) the percutaneous discectomy is being performed for the treatment of lumbago and discogenic pain, in the United States we have adhered to the criteria which was originally developed by the Human Experimentation Committee of The Graduate Hospital in affiliation with the University of Pennsylvania School of Medicine. Our inclusion criteria consist of persistent sciatic pain and failure to respond to conservative therapy, the presence of neurological deficit or positive correlative electromyographic evaluation, positive tension signs, and finally positive correlative CT, MRI, or myelographic findings.

In recent years, we have been able to depend on the combination of CT and MRI studies for the localization of the symptom-producing discs. This has eliminated the need for myelographic studies on a routine basis. The literature is enriched with publications related to psychogenic back pain. The management of the emotional status of the patients with unremitting low back and sciatic pain may be as important as the treatment of their organic disorders. Although some of the more serious and deeply seeded psychiatric disorders of these patients will require specific psychiatric care and counseling, in a clinical setting the majority of these individuals should be treated by clinicians who are involved in their management.

When possible, the operative surgeon should be given the opportunity to examine and treat his patients conservatively in consultation with the referral sources, even if it is for a short period of time. It is during this time frame that both the surgeon and patient will have the opportunity to become acquainted and develop certain mutual respect and rapport. We oppose settings where surgeons are used as technicians, in particular when the diagnosis and treatment plans are made by nonsurgeon participants, and the postoperative follow-up and management are left in the hands of another group of physicians and technicians.

The nature of proposed operative procedures should be discussed, and choices should be reviewed. The possibility of complications of percutaneous lumbar discectomy as compared to conventional methods should be addressed. Although one should not present an unreal optimistic view of the expected results of PLD, certainly a pessimistic attitude would doom the procedure to ultimate failure.

We have found that patient-to-patient contact is an effective way of teaching patients what to expect during the surgery as well as the postoperative period. Patients feel comfortable discussing their pain and difficulties as well as their expected rate of recovery. We encourage these individuals to participate in similar communications with our future surgical candidates. This informal patient-to-patient contact has been helpful in our educational programs and has reduced our patients' level of anxiety which is common in most patients undergoing spine surgery.

The role of conservative therapy for the management of radicular pain due to a protruded disc should not be ignored. The majority of these patients do respond to well-planned conservative therapy. This treatment should include bed rest, nonsteroidal antiinflammatory drugs or short-term steroid therapy. Low doses of antidepressant medication may be used. Educational programs, evaluation of the patient's level of job satisfaction, and the alteration or modification of his or her activities will certainly affect the final outcome of

such treatment. Physical therapy, exercises, and perhaps manipulation treatment should be part of the therapy. However, one should not get locked into a prolonged and unreasonable conservative management. Symptoms associated with intra and perineural fibrosis, secondary to protracted mechanical pressure to the nerve root, may be irreversible. The progression or development of a neurological deficit necessitates the consideration for surgical decompression.

Finally, the patient's level of pain tolerance and the demand for the use of narcotic-based medication should affect the timing for the surgical intervention. The rehabilitation of a drug-dependent patient may be much more complicated than the slim chance of surgical mishap. Emphasis should be placed on the exclusion of individuals with drug dependency. These patients should be enrolled in an effective detoxication program prior to their surgical management. Individuals with psychological disorders, associated with severe anxiety and depression, should have careful assessment and be treated accordingly. Postoperative assessment of individuals involved in compensation claims and litigation disputes continue to pose serious difficulty in proper patient selection for this operative procedure.

Limitations and Advantages

The preoperative diagnostic workup should be directed toward the detection of sequestered discs and bony lateral stenosis. When diagnosed, these conditions should be treated with a conventional laminectomy procedure. The imaging diagnosis of sequestration has been addressed in Chapter 3. However, the presence of severe radicular pain even when the patient is at rest, a large size herniation occupying more than half of the anteroposterior diameter of the spinal canal, and location, shape, and appearance of the extradural defect are criteria which are useful in the diagnosis of a sequestrated disc (5). Patients with signs and symptoms of root compression due to other causes, such as developmental anomalies, primary and metastatic tumors, do not require nor will respond to discectomy. Individuals with long-standing pain and neurological deficits and those with cauda equina syndrome should also be excluded.

The advantages of the percutaneous approach to lumbar discectomy are as follows: there is minimal soft tissue injury. The stripping of the muscles from the spinal processes and laminae, which is required in the course of a laminectomy procedure, poses undesirable morbidity associated with fatigue and backache and demands a lengthy rehabilitation and treatment for the restoration of function. In the course of percutaneous discectomy, the muscles are split and separated with a blunt instrument which eliminates the above unwarranted side effects. The development of intra and perineural fibrosis, due to manipulation, traction of the nerve, and unavoidable epidural bleeding, is not seen when the posterolateral approach is utilized for discectomy. The extrusion of the nuclear fragments through the annular fenestration induced in the course of laminectomy and discectomy procedure has been a cause for concern. An incidence of reherniation as high as 24% has been reported by Atken and Bradford (1). This complication is not encountered following percutaneous lumbar discectomy. The instability induced by zealous bone removal in the course of laminectomy and decompression for posterolateral soft tissue stenosis is eliminated.

Since microlumbar discectomy requires entry into the spinal canal, it carries with it the complications associated with a laminectomy procedure. In our opinion it also poses an additional disadvantage by not providing adequate posterior decompression of the spinal canal. A wide bilateral hemilaminectomy is useful for the treatment of a central or wide base disc protrusions. Since the development of localized stenosis due to disc space narrowing and posterior osteophyte formation is not uncommon following disc herniation treated by laminectomy, adequate posterior decompression will have a tendency to accommodate such stenosis and its associated symptoms postoperatively.

Although the effectiveness of chemonucleolysis for the treatment of uncomplicated disc protrusion has not been challenged, it is fair to state that the enthusiasm for such treatment has been dampened by increasing incidences of complications such as sensitivity reactions, anaphylaxis, chemi-

cal discitis, rapid disc space narrowing, vascular injuries, and severe neurotoxicity (13, 39, 47, 48). The mechanical decompression of the intervertebral disc eliminates the above concerns.

Finally, the cost-effectiveness of percutaneous lumbar discectomy has been significant (17). PLD can be performed on an ambulatory basis. Nevertheless, some of our patients are hospitalized overnight for observation and intravenous antibiotic therapy. All of our patients have been able to become ambulatory shortly following their operative procedure and required only oral pain medication.

Mechanism of Pain Relief

Since the postoperative morbidity of PLD is minimal, a sudden alteration of the intensity of sciatic pain following the surgery becomes strikingly apparent. Currently the decompression of the nerve root by the percutaneous approach is being accomplished by two different techniques. One is aimed toward reduction of the hydrostatic pressure of the intervertebral disc. The other represents a more aggressive approach, aimed not only toward reduction of intradiscal pressure but also the removal of the offending posterolateral nuclear fragments. A simple decompression and reduction of hydrostatic pressure of the intervertebral disc may be achieved by reduction of the nuclear mass through a straight probe inserted dorsolaterally. The reduction of hydrostatic pressure of the intervertebral disc may also be secured by venting of the annulus.

The concept of reducing the volume of the nucleus for the treatment of lumbar radiculopathy associated with disc protrusion is not new. In the course of chemonucleotherapy this goal is achieved through the digestion of protoglycone core protein of the nucleus (49). The inability of chymopapain to digest the collagenized nuclear fragments is held responsible for a number of failures associated with this treatment (50, 52). Certainly one should have no difficulty in removing these fragments by the mechanical means which is accomplished during the course of posterolateral percutaneous lumbar discectomy. When a classic lumbar radiculopathy due to herniated nucleus polposus associated with posterolateral fragments is present, the need for more sophisticated instruments becomes mandatory. Such additional tools include upbiting forceps, backbiting forceps, flexible tip forceps, deflector tube, high negative pressure machine, and discoscope.

Reduction of Hydrostatic Pressure of the Intervertebral Disc

It has been demonstrated that the bulge of the intervertebral disc changes in size during various body positions and following the application of external forces. Virgin (53) has shown that the vertical height of an intervertebral disc is decreased when the disc is subject to an axial compression load. Under such a compression load the annulus bulges outward. Brown et al. (2) demonstrated bulging of the annulus on the side to which the spine is flexed. This was associated with flattening or even slight concavity on the opposite side. Nachemson (34, 35) also reported bulging of the annulus underload associated with increased intradiscal pressure. He has shown that sitting increased the intradiscal pressure by 40%, forward bending and lifting by 100%, and forward flexion and rotation by 400%.

The data suggest that the reduction and perhaps maintaining a low level of intradiscal pressure would be beneficial. In the course of posterolateral discectomy such decompression is achieved by the production of annular fenestration away from the spina canal, therefore reducing the hydrostatic pressure of the nucleus. Unfortunately, medical literature does not provide much information on this interesting concept. To the best of our knowledge Hult (15) was the first surgeon to promote the concept of annular fenestration for the treatment of herniated disc. He reported relief of both low back and sciatic pain in 30 patients following the fenestration of the annulus through an open retroperitoneal approach, stating "If an anterolateral incision is made in the disc, it should be possible to divert the pressure in that direction and thereby prevent it from being transmitted posteriorly".

Markolf et al. (29) were able to demonstrate that the annular fenestration in cadavers was associated with a marked decrease in compressive stiffness and increase in the creep and relaxation rate when the segments were exposed to compression force. Howerver, the extrusion of the nuclear material in young specimens had a tendency to seal the surgical lesion, thus resulting in restoration of the normal compressive behavior. Most of the specimens were obtained from the lower thoracic and upper lumbar region. Only one specimen was from the interspace between the fourth and fifth lumbar segments. One would expect that the older discs with a moderate degree of degeneration and collagenization of the nucleus will show a different behavior pattern. Certainly the thoroughness of discectomy and the application of physiological forces, such as flexion, extension, torsion, and axial rotation may alter the outcome of such a study.

Hampton et al. (9) have reported on the healing potential of a surgically created defect in the annulus of ten dogs. The dogs were sacrificed between 3 to 12 weeks following their surgically induced annular fenestration. The study demonstrated that the defect was eventually filled with a solid plug of fibrous structure presumably from the peripheral tissue. This study supports our clinical observation of CT studies following percutaneous discectomy or laminectomy procedures which have failed to demonstrate the path and location of the intraoperatively induced annular fenestration.

Intraoperatively, we tested the intradiscal pressure of patients prior to and immediately following the lateral decompression and discectomy (20). Following the introduction of a 4.9-mm sheath and prior to fenestration of the annulus by the cutting instrument, a 14-gauge needle containing a slit catheter was introduced into the center of the intervertebral disc. The needle was then withdrawn. One half cubic centimeter of normal saline solution was injected into the disc space, thus creating a liquid media around the tip of the slit catheter. The catheter was then attached to a connecting tube filled with saline solution and a pressure transducer. At this point the intradiscal pressure was considered to be zero. The pressure measuring device was adjusted accordingly. The patient was then instructed to extend his hips and lift his shoulders to permit extension of the lumbar spine. Intradiscal pressure as then measured and recorded. Following the completion of posterolateral decompression and discectomy, the instruments were removed. The measurement of intradiscal pressure was again repeated. In this study we were able to demonstrate a rapid decline of the intradiscal pressure following lateral decompression. The mean rise of intradiscal pressure following the extension of the trunk was 181 mm of mercury. Postoperatively, the pressure dropped to a mean level of 19.4 mm Hg. This difference was statistically significant ($p < 0.01$).

Sakamoto et al. (41) demonstrated up to 40% decline of intradiscal pressure following PLD procedure. The low level of pressure was observed up to 21 months postsurgery in individuals who were tested. These studies demonstrate that adequate annular fenestration with larger instruments and evacuation of nuclear material are equally important in maintaining a low level of intradiscal pressure. The large windowing of the annulus diminishes the chance of early blockage by the retained nuclear fragments. However, it is expected that within a few weeks the defect is sealed, and a low level of hydrostatic pressure of the intervertebral disc is restored.

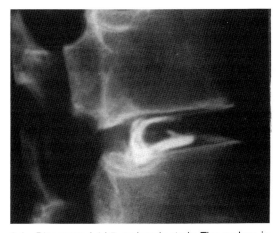

6-1 Discogram L4-L5, cadaveric study. The nucleus is contained and there is no evidence of extravasation of dye.

Extraction of Posterior Nuclear Fragments

The anatomical dissection and study of fresh cadavers are helpful in the understanding of pathophysiology of a normal and herniated intervertebral disc. When normal and intact intervertebral discs are injected with a mixture of methylene blue and renografin-60, one can appreciate the maintenance of the integrity of the annulus fibers as well as the normal appearance of the nucleus (16, 22). The nucleus is centrally located, and there is no evidence of extravasation of the injected opaque substance (Fig. 6-1). The pathological examination of these discs also confirms the presence of intact and homogeneous appearance of the nucleus and the annular fibers (Fig. 6-2).

In contrast to the above, when the degenerative and protruded discs were injected in the same fashion the x-ray study showed the spread of the opaqued material between the torn fibers of the annulus (Fig. 6-3). Although the extravasation of the injected substances to the periannular region of the intervertebral disc or the nerve root sleeves is uncommon, it poses a serious hazard when an incompetent disc is injected with chymopapain or toxic radiographic agents (28) (Fig. 6-4).

The pathological examination of the degenerated intervertebral disc (22, 38) reveals thickening and irregular appearance of the annular fibers associated with both circumferential and radial tears (Fig. 6-5). The migration of the nuclear material between the torn fibers of the annulus may compartmentalize the nucleus (Fig. 6-6). When the fibers of the annulus are only partially torn, a gradually developing disc protrusion is observed. This is associated with an increased anteroposterior and at times the transverse diameter of the intervertebral disc. It has been demonstrated that there is a direct correlation between the narrowing of the intervertebral disc and the size of the annular bulge (16, 22). The size of the protrusion increases when the disc space is narrowed. The degree of the annular protrusion has been measured by A/V index of the spinal units. (Anteroposterior diameter of the intervertebral disc divided by anteroposterior diameter of the vertebral plate below the disc space, Fig. 6-7).

With the advancement of degenerative changes

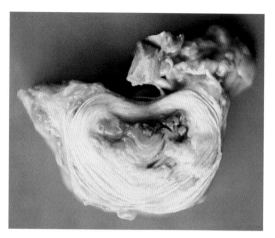

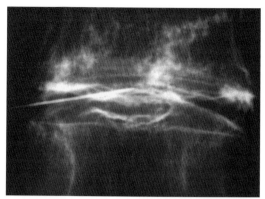

6-2 Gross pathology of the same speciman shown in Figure 6-1. A normal posteriorly positioned nucleus and intact annular fibers are demonstrated.

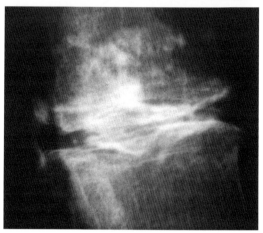

the collagenized nuclear fragments begin to migrate to the periphery and at times are trapped between the torn fibers of annulus, thus producing the CT appearance of a global bulge or protrusion of the intervertebral disc (Fig. 6-8). When the fibers of the annulus are torn and most of its supportive function is eliminated, one can observe a classical radiographic appearance of subligamentous disc herniation. The CT study in this group of patients demonstrates a sudden abrupt soft tissue mass at the herniation site (Fig. 6-9). A small tear of the annulus may allow the expulsion of the nuclear material under the posterior longitudinal ligamentum or its lateral expansion, thus creating a narrow isthmus between the herniation site and the remainder of the nucleus (Fig. 6-10). The presence of the isthmus poses a serious difficulty for ample extraction of the posterior subligamentous disc material, particularly when a straight instrument is being utilized.

These data support the notion that the evacuation of the nuclear material from the center of the latter herniated discs is not possible. An attempt should be made to reach posteriorly to thin out the partially torn annular fibers, thus allowing the removal of the nuclear fragments or facilitating their central migration.

6-3 Discogram L4-L5 in a 50-year-old male. Cadaveric study. The torn annular fibers have allowed the peripheral extravasation of the opaque material.

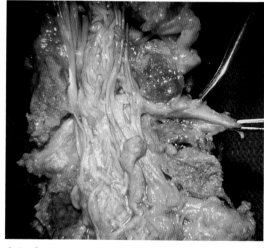

6-4 Cadaveric study. The injected mixture of methylene blue and opaque material has penetrated the dural sheath around the nerve root in a retrograde fashion.

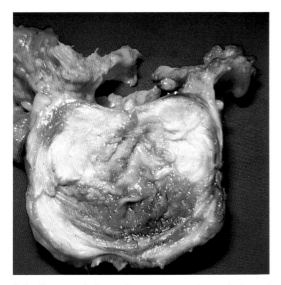

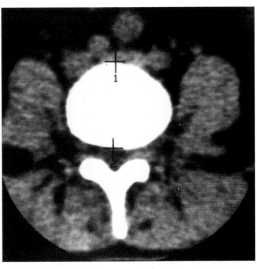

6-5 Gross pathology of speciman 3 shows thickened irregular and torn annular fibers allowing the extravasation of dye.

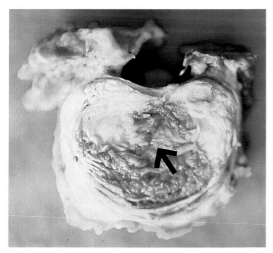

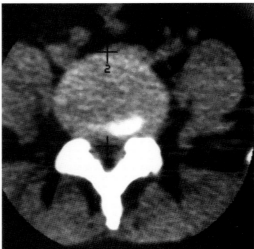

6-7 A/V index of the spinal unit.

6-6 Degenerative compartmentalization of the nucleus.

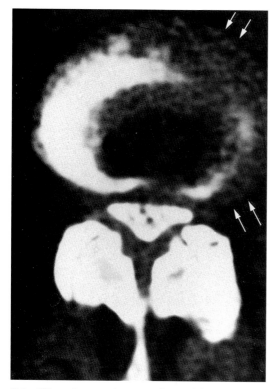

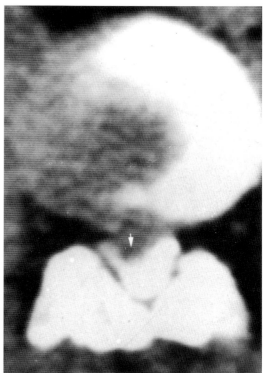

6-8 CT myelogram demonstrating a global bulge of a degenerated intervertebral disc.

6-9 CT myelogram of herniated nucleus pulposus.

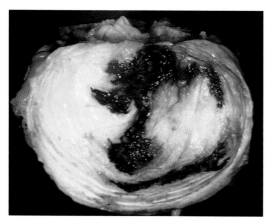

6-10 Cadaveric study. The torn inverted annular fibers are connecting the two compartments of the nucleus via a narrow isthmus.

Needle Insertion

The proper insertion and positioning of the needle is the most important initial step in a satisfactory completion of posterolateral percutaneous lumbar discectomy. This technique permits precisional introduction of the subsequent instruments. It also allows the cannulated trocar and the inserted sheath to follow the exact path of the anesthetic column. The insertion of a blunt trocar without the guide wire increases the chance of soft tissue injury and the development of psoas hematoma.

With the patient in a prone position the C-arm is maneuvered to provide a true lateral image of the lower lumbar segments and the sacrum. The visualization of the sacrum will assure the proper counting and correct selection of the surgical site. The point of entry is approximately 10 cm from the midline. In obese patients with abundant subcutaneous adipose tissue a further distance from the midline may have to be chosen. We prefer to introduce the instruments from the symptomatic side. If right sciatic pain is present the needle is inserted 10 cm from the midline on the right side of the patient and vice versa. A preoperative abdominal CT through the herniation site allows the surgeon to select the point of entry, thus avoiding a far lateral insertion which may violate the abdominal cavity (Fig. 6-11). One has to make certain that the instruments are well placed in the sacrospinalis, quadratus lumbrum, and psoas major

muscles (Fig. 6-12). The angle of the needle insertion in reference to the horizontal plane may be measured from the same abdominal CT. When the needle is inserted too close to the midline it directs the open end of the subsequently introduced working sheath somewhat laterally. However, when the point of entry is approximately 10 cm from the midline the distal extremity of the sheath is pointed medially and posteriorly. This allows better access to the posterior half of the intervertebral disc.

During the needle insertion the surgeon should rely on eye-hand coordination (25). As soon as the tip of the inserted needle meets with resistance, it should be viewed in the lateral x-ray projection. If posterior positioning is demonstrated, the needle is then withdrawn and reinserted in an increased angle in reference to the horizontal plane (Fig. 6-13). In contrast, if no resistance is encountered following several centimeters of penetration, the position should be checked again in the lateral view. The failure to meet with resistance is most likely due to a vertical insertion and should be corrected accordingly (Fig. 6-14).

If the preoperative abdominal CT through the herniated site has not been obtained and the angle for the introduction of the needle has not been determined, it is always safer to start with a lesser angle than a vertical insertion. Ideally, one would like to view the tip of the needle in the lateral x-ray projection at the posterolateral corner of the inter-

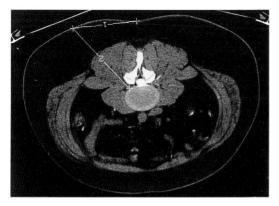

6-11 Preoperative abdominal CT demonstrates the desirable angle of introduction of the needle from a distance of 10 cm from the midline.

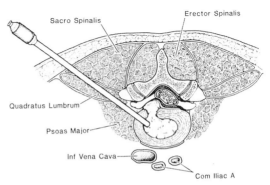

6-12 Cross-section of the surgical site.

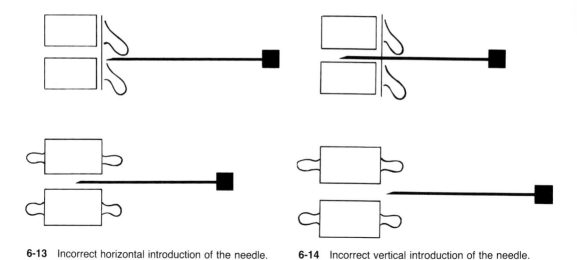

6-13   Incorrect horizontal introduction of the needle.

6-14   Incorrect vertical introduction of the needle.

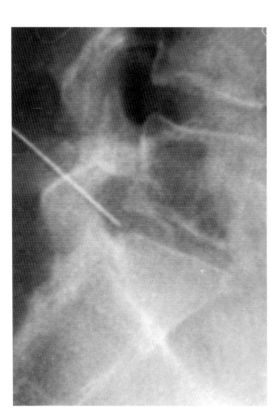

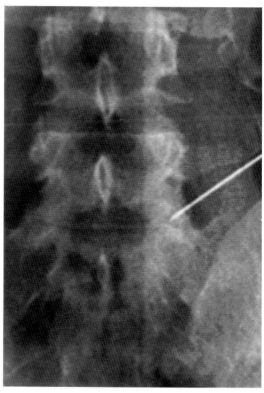

6-15   Interoperative C-arm imaging in the lateral projection. The tip of the needle is seen on posterior border of the intervertebral disc.

6-16   The AP projection of the needle, insertion shown in Figure 6-15. The tip of the needle is viewed in alignment with a line drawn at midpart of the pedicle of the superior and inferior vertebrae.

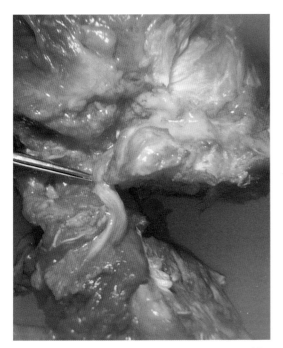

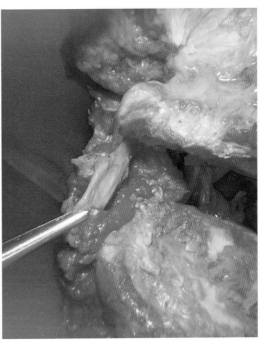

6-17 Anatomical speciman showing the departure of the spinal nerve from the foramina, its descent and position anterior to the transverse process.

6-18 Another view of speciman shown in Figure 6-17. The psoas muscle fibers are seen between the spinal nerve and the annulus.

vertebral disc or slightly anterior to it (Fig. 6-15). The visualization of the needle tip in the AP projection is as important as it is in the lateral view. The tip of the needle should be placed just lateral to the proximal articular process of the inferior vertebrae. Thus, in the AP projection the tip of the needle is viewed in alignment with the midportion of the pedicles or slightly lateral to it (Fig. 6-16).

As soon as the spinal nerve departs from the foramina, it moves anteriorly, distally, and laterally. It is then positioned anterior to the transverse process within the fibers of psoas muscle (Fig. 6-17 and 6-18). In the absence of degenerative changes of the facets joints and posterior osteophytosis there is some mobility of the spinal nerve at this region. Only the origin of the spinal nerve which is extended from the foramina across the annulus to the superior border of the transverse process is subject to penetration and injury.

Generally, there is ample space in the triangular working zone (18, 20, 25) for the introduction of the instruments. The triangular working zone is

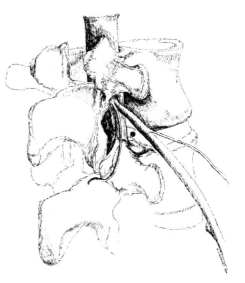

6-19 The *solid circle* shows the correct position of the tip of the needle in the triangular working zone (proximal vertebral plate inferiorly, the articular process of the lower segment posteriorly, and the spinal nerve anteriorly).

bordered by the proximal vertebral plate of the lower lumbar segment inferiorly, the proximal articular process of the lower segment posteriorly, and the spinal nerve anteriorly (Fig. 6-19). Due to anatomical variation one may encounter contact with the spinal nerve while attempting to achieve the above positioning. In this event the needle may have to be relocated more anteriorly. When it is possible the needle should be inserted parallel to the vertebral plates in order to prevent contact between the inserted instruments and the vertebral plates, thus providing better access to the intervertebral disc and the herniated site.

Annular Fenestration

Currently the entry into the intervertebral discs for the introduction of the working sheath and instruments is accomplished by two methods: gradual dilatation or a one-step entry utilizing the circular cutting instruments. In the gradual dilatation method (42, 43, 51) first a spinal needle with a removable hub is introduced dorsolaterally into the annulus. This step is followed by the introduction of several larger tubes which are inserted in succession (Fig. 6-20).

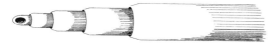

6-20 The gradual dilatation of the annulus over the inserted needle.

This method appears to have two distinct disadvantages. The introduction of the larger cannula into an intact annulus particularly in a young subject is rather difficult, and it may cause the migration of the smaller inner cannula and its entry into the abdominal cavity. This system also will have a tendency to position the open end of the working sheath at the center of the disc during the inception of the procedure. From the center of the disc it is rather difficult to reach the posterior fragments. In contrast, when the annulus is windowed, as the working sheath is resting on the outer surface of the annulus, the surgeon has the

capability of reaching and evacuating such fragments adjacent to the open extremity of the inserted sheath on the dorsolateral aspect of the intervertebral disc adjacent to the herniation site. This step is followed by gradual engagement of the cannula into the annulus, thus allowing further evacuation with the straight and curved forceps.

The size of the annular fenestration appears to be an important factor affecting the final outcome of percutaneous lumbar discectomy. Such an opening may allow the continuous decompression and reduction of the posterior nuclear fragments following the termination of the PLD procedure. For this reason, the circular fenestration of the annulus is preferred.

There has been legitimate concern among spinal surgeons about the feasibility of the introduction of large instruments through the posterolateral approach. The fear of causing neural injury has encouraged the development and utilization of small caliber automated instruments (37) which allow only the cannulization and minimal central evacuation of the intervertebral disc. There is no foundation for such conservatism. The anatomical studies conducted in our center (20) and a subsequent study by Shepperd (44, 45) have demonstrated that there is ample space in the previously described triangular working zone which can accommodate larger instruments up to 8 to 9 mm in diameter.

The larger fenestration of the annulus not only allows the continuous decompression but it also provides room for the introduction of the special instruments which are necessary for adequate evacuation. Originally we were using a 2.5-mm cutting instrument to penetrate the annulus. As we gained experience, we were able to introduce larger diameter instruments with relative safety. Although the small caliber sheath and cutting instruments are still available, we rarely find them necessary or useful.

At the present time we are utilizing a cutting instrument with an outer diameter of 4.5 mm. However, the majority of narrowed disc spaces which do not allow the introduction of the 4.5-mm cutter most often demonstrate posterior and posterolateral osteophytosis and are not a proper choice for percutaneous lumbar discectomy.

The fenestration of the annulus is usually associated with some pain and discomfort which may require the systemic use of analgesics by the anesthesiologist. The pain arising from this step of the operation is attributed either to pain receptor nerve fibers in the expansion of the posterior longitudinal ligamentum or is due to the increase of intradiscal pressure when the surgeon applies pressure on the annulus. The reproduction of the patient's sciatic pain when the annulus is compressed by the blunt trocar may have diagnostic validity. The compression of the annulus of a normal intervertebral disc with a blunt end instrument should not cause radicular pain.

For a rapid fenestration of the annulus and the reduction of intradiscal pressure the surgeon should start with the small cutting instrument which is then followed with the 4.5 circular cutter.

How to Avoid Spinal Nerve Injury

Entrapment of the spinal nerve under the inserted sheath is unlikely and is extremely painful. With an apprehensive patient the surgeon should first evaluate the position of the sheath via C-arm imaging to make certain that the distal extremity of the working sheath is correctly positioned in both the AP and lateral projection.

A simple needle testing is useful not only for centering the sheath on the annulus but to make certain that the spinal nerve is not in the path of the inserted sheath. A sharp needle is used, and the annulus is perforated repeatedly. In the absence of nerve root entrapment the tip of the needle will enter the annulus with no major pain or discomfort. In contrast, if the nerve is in the path of the sheath the patient will experience servere radicular pain.

The direct visualization of the annulus with the discoscope is extremely helpful, particularly with patients of a low pain threshold. While the surgeon is holding the sheath against the annulus the 0- or 30°-angle scope is introduced. The suction irrigation system is established in a routine fashion. In the absence of nerve entrapment the annulus has a smooth homogenous appearance; however, at times, superficial veins crossing its surface are seen (see Operative Technique page 85).

Finally the pattern of distribution of the radicular pain as expressed by the patient assists the surgeon to rule out nerve root entrapment. The dermatomal distribution of radicular pain arising from the L5 root compression secondary to herniated disc at L4–L5 differs from the irritation of the L4 spinal nerve which may have been impinged by the instruments inserted dorsolaterally into L4–L5 intervertebral disc in the course of percutaneous discectomy.

Evacuation

The principles which have been practiced for disc extraction following a laminectomy procedure are applicable to percutaneous lumbar discectomy. The effectiveness of central evacuation is thought to be secondary to the reduction of volume of nucleus, which in turn may cause the reduction of the herniation and ultimately the relief of sciatic pain. The central decompression of an intervertebral disc is rather simple. It is achieved by the introduction of a straight tube into the center of the disc space. The removal of nuclear material is then achieved either with forceps or an automated instrument (10–12, 37).

The challenge of posterolateral percutaneous discectomy lies in the capability of reaching posteriorly and evacuating the offending nuclear fragments. The evacuation of the nucleus is not complete without an attempt by the operative surgeon to remove the posteriorly lodged fragments. Occasionally, the partially torn annular fibers must be thinned out by angled forceps. Then, the fragments are pulled in by forced suction and angled forceps.

The deflector tube allows approximately 40° of angulation of the distal extremity of the flexible forceps. As the deflector tube is advanced or partially withdrawn, the various parts of the annulus, consisting of right and left posterolateral and midline protrusions, are reached and evacuated. Ring curets also are available and should be used to free the loose fragments.

The design of the instruments permits only 2 cm of penetration of the instruments behind the tip of the inserted sheath. Invariably, it is desirable to advance the sheath into the annulus to achieve better central and peripheral evacuation. Great care should be exercised not to remove or disturb the intact anterior or lateral annular structures. Such a practice will cause a more rapid narrowing and the collapse of the height of the intervertebral disc.

Negative Pressure

In our early clinical research we have reported the potential benefit of forced suction in the field of percutaneous lumbar discectomy (21). Such negative pressure is capable of bringing the loose nuclear material into the path of the inserted sheath and facilitates their evacuation. Our original cadaveric studies gave us confidence in the safety of the introduction of high negative pressure into the intervertebral disc. Our subsequent utilization of negtive pressure, as high as 29 inches of mercury in more than 150 patients, has proven its safety and usefulness.

The wall suctions, which are available in the operating room, do not produce adequate negative pressure in the intervertebral disc. We have employed a 50-cc syringe to create high negative pressure. Currently, we are working with negative pressure pumps which are used in liposuction procedures.

C-Arm Imaging

Precise visualization of the lumbar segments and the intervertebral discs with the C-arm is essential. In order to view the intervertebral discs in the lateral projection the x-ray beams should be directed parallel to the vertebral plates. In the AP view it is important to make certain that the spinal process is in the midline and pedicles are well-visualized and symmetrical. With an obese patient, one may have difficulty visualizing the lower lumbar segments. These particular patients should be seen in the Radiology Department prior to surgery to make sure that the intraoperative fluoroscopy is possible.

One should make certain that the draping of the C-arm will not interfere with its rotation and will allow reproducible imaging throughout the surgery. Sterile plastic sheaths are now available and can be used for draping.

Positioning of the Patient

Percutaneous lumbar discectomy can be performed with the patient either in a prone or lateral position (11, 12). Surgeons who have performed chemonucleotherapy in the lateral position may feel more comfortable with side positioning. However, we have abandoned the lateral positioning for three reasons. Patients appear to be more secure in the prone position. If they rotate or move their trunk, the repositioning takes place automatically as the patient relaxes. To secure the patient in a side position is more time-consuming than the prone. Finally, when the biportal approach is desired for a discoscopy or arthrodesis, the patient must be maintained in the prone position.

One may utilize rolled sheets on the side of the patient. The rolls are extended from the iliac crest to the side of the chest wall. The disadvantage of the rolled sheets is that it does not provide adequate flexion and flattening of the lumbar spine, which is of great importance for L5-S1 discectomy. Furthermore, the sheets are unstable and invariably roll out from under the patient. Adjustable radiolucent frames are now available. They provide adequate flexion of the hip joints while reducing the pressure on the abdominal cavity (Fig. 6-21). The maximum height of the bolster at the midportion is 7 inches, and it gradually tapers down to 2½ inches.

It is desirable to keep the patient's flexed knees slightly off the table top. This provides slight traction and tilt of the pelvis by flexing the OR table just distal to the lower extremity of the adjustable frame. This is of particular importance when attempting L5-S1 discectomy. A slight tilt of the pelvis to the side while the patient is in prone position is also possible. The latter is helpful in clearing the iliac crest away from the path of the inserted instruments.

The majority of operating rooms are equipped with radiolucent tables. The radiolucent extensions, which are attached to the operating room tables, are also available. Up-to-date fracture tables are suitable for percutaneous discectomy.

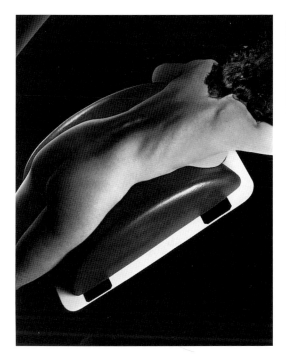

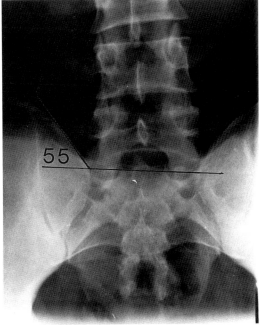

6-21 Adjustable radiolucent frame allows the reduction of the lumbar lordosis and diminishes the pressure on the abdomen.

6-22 AP x-ray of the pelvis showing a prominent iliac spine and acute angle between the medial extremity of the iliac crest and the proximal plate of the sacrum.

When the patient is properly positioned, the table is tilted to bring the lumbar spine of the patient into a horizontal plane. This allows proper C-arm imaging.

Preoperative Imaging

Plane radiographic evaluation of the lumbar spine is helpful in both diagnosis and surgical planning of patients with herniated lumbar discs. In most instances a limited screening x-ray study in AP and lateral projection is adequate. If there is a question of mechanical instability, the dynamic x-rays in flexion and extension and also side bending views should be obtained. The determination of accessibility of a given intervertebral disc to the percutaneous posterolateral discectomy is important in the preoperative planning particularly when attempting L5-S1 discectomy. Both AP and lateral x-ray films will provide information in this regard.

An attempt should be made to keep the iliac crests on the same plane when exposing a lateral x-ray film from the lumbosacral articulation. In most instances the iliac crest is in alignment with the L4-L5 disc interspace. Generally when the iliac crest is above the L4-L5 disc, the access to and evacuation of a herniated disc at L5-S1 are difficult. The shape of the iliac crest as visualized in the AP x-ray projection provides more specific information regarding the approachability of L5-S1 disc. The evacuation of the L5-S1 discs in individuals with a prominent iliac spine who demonstrate an acute angle between the medial extremity of the iliac crest and proximal plate of the sacrum is usually difficult (Fig. 6-22). In contrast, when the iliac crest is rather flat and the above angle is reduced one has less difficulty approaching the L5-S1 intervertebral disc (Fig. 6-23). When the patient has an unusually wide transverse process of L5 in conjunction with a high iliac crest, the introduction of the instruments to L5-S1 becomes more cumbersome.

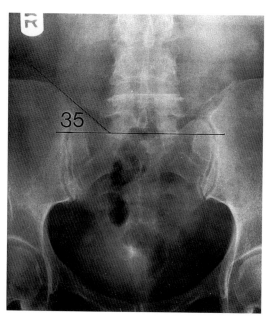

6-23 AP x-ray of the pelvis as in Figure 6-22. The iliac crest is at the level of L4-L5 disc space; however, the iliac spine is less prominent.

The plane radiographs should also be examined for detection of developmental abnormalities and bone lesions. The narrowing of a single intervertebral disc and the presence of posterior osteophytes which correlates with the patient's dermatomal radicular pain and the neurological findings are suggestive of spinal stenosis and bulging disc which may be responsible for the patient's symptoms.

MRI, CT, and Myelography

At this state of the art the MRI is the most useful initial screening test prior to surgical intervention. The noninvasive nature of this study as well as the wealth of information that it provides have made it quite appealing to both patient and physician. When a better visualization of the herniated sight in axial projection is desired, the CT study from the suspected level will provide additional needed information prior to the surgical intervention. The MRI is rapidly eliminating the need for routine preoperative myelography for diagnostic purposes.

Selective Discography and Pain Provocative Testing

Lindblom (26) is credited with the introduction of discography as a tool for the diagnosis of painful disc syndrome. The necessity and reliability of discography have been controversial in both the diagnosis and treatment of low back pain with or without radiculopathy. The literature is enriched with both favorable (3, 8, 36, 46) as well as critical reports (6, 14) on this subject.

In recent years advanced technology such as MR imaging and CT discography has enhanced our capability of visualizing the internal structures of the intervertebral disc. The CT and MR study of the lumbar spine has enabled us to diagnose the lateral stenosis as well as foraminal and the extraforaminal disc herniations which was not possible with the commonly used myelographic evaluation. The significant contribution of these diagnostic tools also has created unavoidable confusion which has added further burden in decision making as related to the detection of the symptom-producing site. The abnormal extradural soft tissue prominences are often present and reported in multiple levels. The terms of bulging annulus, bulging disc, herniated disc, protruded disc, etc. are used interchangeably by radiologists to describe these findings and therefore recommending further clinical correlation. Unfortunately due to anatomical variation, the accurate diagnosis of the exact level of lumbar root compression by the clinical examination even when the neurological deficit is present is not always possible. The clinical invariably is in need of additional objective support to substantiate his clinical judgement and his surgical management. Under these circumstances, selective discography and disc expansion testing may provide valuable information. However, in a great majority of patients one should be able to enter into an accurate diagnosis of the level of root compression utilizing the clinical findings and the available technology, namely, MRI, CT, and myelography. A routine indiscriminate discography on multiple levels when the above studies have been negative is uninformative and rarely necessary.

The information that is obtained in the course of discography, namely, the amount of fluid which is accepted by a given disc, the radiographic appearance, and the pain reproduction are reported to be helpful in isolating the pain-producing intervertebral discs. The pressure under which the normal saline or opaque material is injected into the disc also may affect the radiographic appearance of the study (19). An intact intervertebral disc is capable of withstanding a considerable amount of internal load. However, a degenerated and partially torn annulus may be further damaged or ruptured under undue pressure. The radiographic appearance of the normal and abnormal discograms with or without an accompanying CT evaluation as well as the classification of CT discography has been well-described (30, 40). The MR imaging also has been helpful in the diagnosis of degenerative changes of the intervertebral disc and the annular insufficiency. The pain reproduced following discography or disc distention testing remains the unique property of this study. When the pain reproduction is associated with an abnormal discogram, CT or MRI study, the diagnosis of the symptom-producing level becomes more evident.

MacMillan et al. (28) performed 130 lumbar discograms in 21 randomly selected fresh cadavers. The lumbar segments were then removed, dissected and studied. It was demonstrated that leakage of the injected fluid to the periannular region was not uncommon. Fifteen of the above intervertebral discs were incompetent. Although thick adhesions between the posterior longitudinal ligament and posterior dura were observed (Fig. 6-24), none of the specimens showed the extravasation of the dye into the subarachnoid space through this route. The most common path of communication was lateral to the posterior longitudinal ligament into the epidural space. The injected agent descended around the spinal nerve in three instances; it penetrated the dural sleeve of the nerve root in retrograde fashion in one (Fig. 6-4). It was concluded that a significant risk exists when neurotoxic material is injected into an incompetent intervertebral disc. Such material may come in contact with the neural tissue or on a rare occasion extravasation to the subarachnoid space may occur. When performing discography, one should consider less toxic radiopaque agents which are now available for myelographic examination. The pain experienced during or following

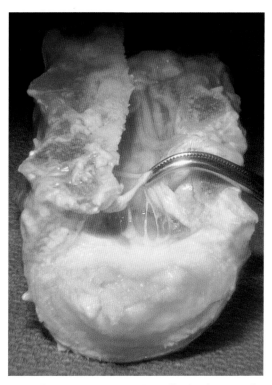

6-24 Cadaveric study showing adhesion between the posterior dura and posterior longitudinal ligament.

injection of the neurotoxic material into an incompetent intervertebral disc can be explained on the basis of irritation of one or more nerve roots. Thus, the diagnostic validity of pain reproduction during discography in the setting of an incompetent disc remains questionable. However, recreation of symptomatic pain produced by injection of a disc proven competent by discography remains a significant contribution of discography in the diagnosis of painful disc syndrome.

Our indications for selective discography and disc distention testing are as follows:
1. Inability to secure MRI, CT, or myelography or when the studies are not optimal or obtainable due to excessive obesity, allergies, claustrophobia, or metallic implants
2. Equivocal radiological report of findings which understates or overdescribes the findings in multiple levels
3. The evaluation of the intervertebral disc adjacent to the segment which is under consideration for fusion

4. The determination of an annular or ligamentous tear following trauma in a young individual
   who exhibited persistent pain, rigidity, and
   limitation of mobility and has failed conservative therapy
5. Diagnosis of sequestration in geographic areas
   where adequate MR or CT imaging is not
   available

Instruments

The arsenals of instrumentation for percutaneous
lumbar discectomy have been growing rapidly.
However, our basic manual instruments have continued to be effective and useful.

Standard Manual Instruments

The available spinal kit (Fig. 6-25) contains the
following: an 18-gauge spinal needle which is 5
inches in length, Kirschner wire, cannulated trocar
with an external diameter of 4.5 mm and a length
of 19 cm, working sheath with an external diameter of 6.5 mm and an internal diameter of 4.9 mm
and a length of 16 cm, and two sizes of circular
cutting instruments having 3- and 4.5-mm cutting
ends.

The length of the cutting instruments are 18 cm,
thus allowing only 2 cm of penetration into the
intervertebral disc as the working sheath rests
against the annulus. The cutting instruments have
a permanently attached Luer Lok fitting which acts
as a handle when attempting entry into the intervertebral disc. This can also be used for the introduction of forced suction in the course of the
surgical procedure. A deflector tube is also provided and has a removable Luer Lok fitting which
can be used for introduction of negative pressure
directed posteriorly. The collar of the deflector
tube is marked to indicate the position of the open
end of the instrument when it is fully inserted into
the working sheath. A flexible tip forceps which is
used in conjunction with the deflector tube allows
40 ° dorsal angulation following its full insertion
(Fig. 6-26). Two straight forceps with 3-mm and
4-mm cups and an angle forceps with a 2-mm cup
are also part of the basic instrument set. The design

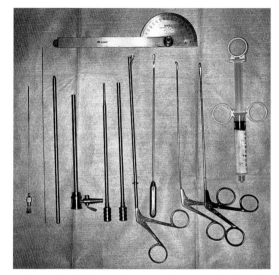

6-25 Spinal kit from left to right: 18-gauge spinal needle, guide wire, cannulated trocar, working sheath with the attached adaptor, small circular cutter, large circular cutter, deflector tube and flexible forceps, curet, upbiting forceps, straight forceps, syringe and Xylocaine solution. Top shows goniometer.

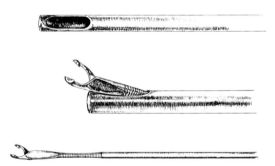

6-26 The deflector tube and flexible tip forceps.

of the instruments does not permit more than 2 cm
penetration beyond the open end of the working
sheath for safety purposes. The flexible tip forceps
is longer and should be used only in conjunction
with the defector tube. Ring curets, backbiting
forceps, and magnetic retrieval rods are also currently available.

Auxiliary Instruments

Power cutting instruments which are currently used in the course of surgical arthroscopy have been modified for disc extraction (Figs. 6-27 and 6-28). These instruments allow the simultaneous cutting, irrigation, and extraction of the nuclear fragments. They allow more rapid withdrawal of the nuclear material than the manual instruments.

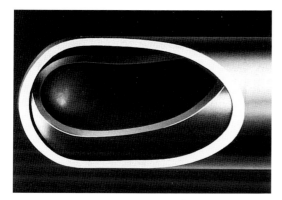

6-27 The distal extremity of powered cutting instrument.

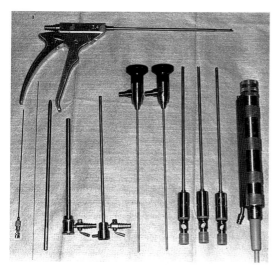

6-28 *Top:* Suction punch forceps. *Bottom from left to right:* 18-gauge needle, guide wire, cannulated trocar, working sheath, the internal sheath for discoscopy or utilization of simultaneous cutting and irrigation system, various angle discoscopes, three cutting instruments, handle for powered blades.

A drop lock adaptor which fits snugly to the end of the working sheath has to be utilized in conjunction with the power cutting instruments. The inflow of saline solution is provided by a valve on the drop lock adaptor. The severed pieces of the nuclear material are irrigated and removed through the space provided inside the tube of the cutting blade and collected. Minimal negative pressure is required when powered instruments are used. Various shapes of cutting instruments are available. However, the full radius blade is most commonly used. The automated instruments are most useful for rapid evacuation of the nuclear material in young individuals. However, in older discs where the collagenization of the nucleus has taken place it may be necessary to use the manual tools for the extraction of such fragments.

Discoscope

Biportal discoscopy has been advocated and described by Schreiber et al. (42, 43). Although such an approach may be useful and necessary for the purpose of performing percutaneous interbody fusion, we feel that it increases the operative time, radiation exposure, the possibility for complications, and overall morbidity of the procedure.

We have used discoscopy intermittently with our manual and power-driven instruments through a single port. Our prototype uniportal discoscope provides for the inflow and outflow of normal saline solution through the same assembly which fits inside of the working sheath and the drop lock adaptor. With the availability of newer flexible small caliber fiberoptics, further improvement in our existing working scope is anticipated, and its common use for discectomy may become a reality.

Operative Technique

To diminish the chance of infection and its serious consequences the percutaneous discectomy should be performed in the operating room under a strict sterile environment. We use a prophylactic antibiotic for 24 hours in all of our patients. The first dose is given in the operating room prior to the surgery. This is followed by two additional doses provided every eight hours.

Our preference is to perform this procedure with the patient in the prone position. When the patient is in the lateral position, any movement or rotation of the trunk will alter the ability to obtain a reproducible x-ray imaging. However, proper repositioning of the patient is done with ease when the patient is placed in the prone.

The patient is placed in a radiolucent adjustable frame which provides for freedom of the abdomen and flattens the lumbosacral angle (Fig. 6-21). The proper positioning is of particular importance for the L5-S1 disc extraction. The C-arm is positioned and covered by sterile plastic or cloth sheet. One should make certain that the sterile cover will not interfere with the free rotation of the C-arm. For better visualization of the L5-S1 disc space a slight tilt of the C-arm may be necessary. The skin preparation and draping is similar to any open procedure. Care should be exercised not to place metallic clips in the path of the surgical site.

The iliac crest and spinal processes are identified and marked accordingly. In most individuals one can palpate the lateral extension of the paraspinal muscles as a reference point prior to the needle insertion. The desirable site for the needle insertion may be predetermined by CT study prior to the surgery (Fig. 6-11). By placing a metallic marker on the skin and floroscopic control the relation of the iliac crest to the surgical site in the anteroposterior projection is then identified.

The intraoperative communication with the patient is essential. The patients should not be heavily sedated nor should general anesthesia be utilized. Skin, subcutaneous tissue, fascia, and muscle layers are infiltrated with 1% Xylocaine solution. To diminish muscular bleeding, the Xylocaine solution containing epinephrine is injected into the muscle layers. In order to prevent an anesthetic block of the spinal nerve and the development of neural injury by the inserted instruments, one should avoid the periannular infiltration of the local anesthetics.

The 18-gauge needle is then inserted from a distance of approximately 9 or 10 cm from the midline and directed toward the annulus. The proper positioning of the tip of the needle prior to its insertion into the annular fibers should be

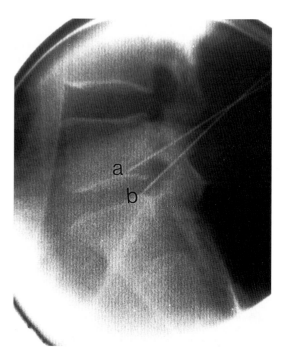

6-29 *(a)* Incorrect position of the needle. *(b)* Correct position.

documented radiographically. The assessment of the correct position of the tip of the needle in the triangular working zone by floroscopic examination when the needle has been introduced into the annular fibers is rather difficult. When the needle is properly positioned its tip is seen in the lateral view adjacent to the posterior border of the disc space or slightly lateral to it. In the AP projection the tip of the needle should be visualized on the line or slightly lateral to the line which is drawn between the midpart of the pedicles of the vertebrae above and below the disc space (Figs. 6-15 and 6-16). At times one can use an unacceptable inserted needle as a guide for the introduction of the next needle (Fig. 6-29).

At this time the stylet of the needle is withdrawn and replaced by a guide wire. In order to secure the wire and prevent it from becoming dislodged when the needle is being extracted, the tip of the wire is engaged in the annular fibers for a distance of 4 to 5 mm. The removal of the needle is accomplished by a slow rotary movement, thus leaving the guide wire in position. A small incision is made around

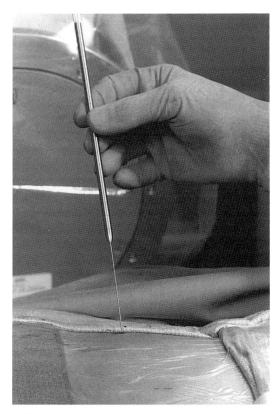

6-30 The introduction of the cannulated trocar over the guide wire.

the guide wire to allow the introduction of the larger instruments. The cannulated trocar is placed over the wire and directed toward the annulus (Fig. 6-30) with a firm rotary movement. The trocar follows the column of previously injected local anesthetics with precision. A right-handed surgeon should maintain downward pressure of the cannulated trocar with the left hand while using the right hand to rotate and further advance the instrument. A certain amount of resistance is encountered when the trocar is being passed through the fascia.

It is advisable to disengage the tip of the guide wire from the annulus or withdraw it as soon as the direction and position of the cannulated trocar in the paraspinal muscles is firmly established. Inevitably at times the trocar is angulated while it is being inserted, and therefore it does not follow the exact path of the inserted guide wire. In this case

the inserted trocar will cause the wire to bend or even break, thus creating difficulty for its extraction.

When the needle is properly inserted the fixation of the spinal nerve against the annulus by the inserted guide wire is rare, and the surgeon is alerted by the strong protest of pain by the patient. In this event the withdrawal of the guide wire prior to full insertion of the cannulated trocar as described above will allow the blunt end of the trocar to bypass the spinal nerve and attain its proper position on the annulus (Fig. 6-31).

The standard working sheath with an internal diameter of 4.9 mm is then positioned over the cannulated trocar and directed toward the annulus. We have abandoned the use of smaller or larger caliber working sheaths for routine discectomies. The inserted trocar should be held firmly against the annulus and not withdrawn until the working sheath is fully inserted and its correct position is documented radiographically. When the sheath is fully inserted the round end of the trocar is no longer seen in the AP and lateral floroscopic examination. Since there is a 3 cm difference between the length of the inserted sheath and the trocar, the surgeon is able to determine whether or not the sheath has been fully inserted.

As the working sheath is firmly held against the annulus, a needle testing is conducted. The insertion of a sharp needle into the annulus by walking inside the open end of the sheath is helpful in centering the sheath on the annular fibers prior to the use of the cutting instruments. This test is also used to differentiate between the radicular pain which is generated by increased intradiscal pressure due to compression of the annulus by the instruments and the nerve root entrapment. When the spinal nerve is not in the path of the inserted sheath the sharp point of the 20-gauge needle penetrates the annulus with no major pain or difficulty. However, the needling of the spinal nerve is extremely painful. We have used the discoscope for visualization and inspection of the annulus prior to the use of circular cutting instruments and entry to the disc space. The annulus usually has a smooth reddish surface (Fig. 32A). At times small branches of the lumbar vein crossing the annulus at the sight of the intended fenestration is seen (Fig. 6-32B). Slight bleeding pro-

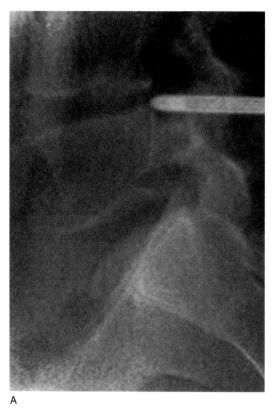
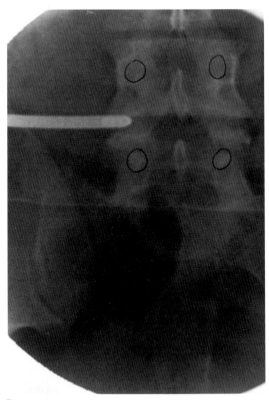

A   B

6-31   *(A)* Proper position of the trocar on the annulus in the lateral projection. *(B)* The correct position of the trocar on the annulus in the AP projection. The tip of the trocar is in alignment with a line drawn between the midpart of the pedicle of the proximal and distal segments.

duced by the severance of the annulus should be of no concern. The bleeding is usually controlled by the engagement of the distal end of the working sheath into the annular fibers by firm rotary and downward pressure for a distance of 2 or 3 mm. Occasionally a thin layer of fatty tissue obstructs the proper inspection of the annulus (Fig. 6-32 C). In this case a moist cottonoid is used, and the adipose tissue is rubbed off the annular surface, thus allowing its visualization. Although it is not recommended, one can visualize the spinal nerve by tilting the cannula slightly cephalad and anteriorly (Fig. 6-32 D)

The superficial layer of the annulus and the lateral expansion of the posterior longitudinal ligament contain sensory nerve fibers (Chapter 2). Prior to fenestration of the annulus the systemic use of analgesics by the anesthesiologist may be deemed necessary. The infiltration of the annular fibers with local anesthetics in a young individual is usually difficult. However, a forceful injection of less than 0.5 cc of Xylocaine solution into the annular fibers followed by the withdrawal of the needle may result in subsequent leakage of the injected solution into the surface of the annulus, thus providing topical anesthesia. At times the placement of a cottonoid, which has been saturated in Xylocaine solution, on the annulus will provide adequately needed topical anesthesia.

The fenestration of the annulus is accomplished first with the smaller circular cutting instrument which is followed with the introduction of the larger cutter. Since the working sheath is resting on the annulus, it does not permit the cutting instruments to penetrate the disc space more than 2 cm. This represents a safety feature provided by the design in order to avoid deep penetration of the

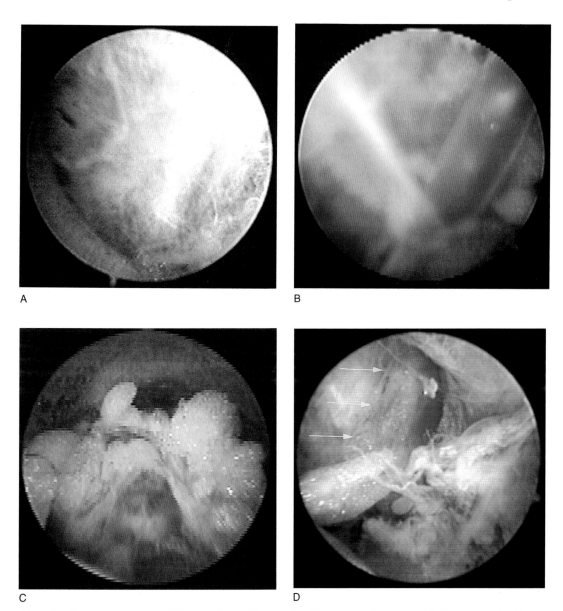

A

B

C

D

6-32 *(A)* Normal appearance of the annulus in disco-scopic examination. *(B)* A superficial vein is noted cross-ing the annulus. *(C)* Loose fatty tissue covering the an-nulus. *(D)* Arthroscopic view of the spinal nerve.

cutting instruments. This measure prevents seri-ous bowl or vascular injuries. The cutting instru-ments may be left in position as a guide when the working sheath is advanced with firm rotary movement and is engaged into the annulus for a distance not more than 2 or 3 mm. This prevents periannular migration of the working sheath dur-ing evacuation.

Following the removal of the circular cutter the surgeon must hold the working sheath with one hand while using the opposite hand for the intro-duction of the instruments and the removal of disc fragments. The surgeon should make a mental note of the numerical markers on the outer surface of the working sheath which indicates its depth of penetration. Although the central migration of the

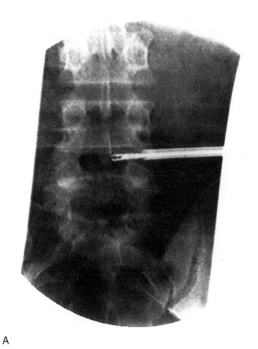

A

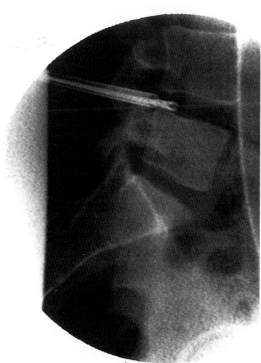

B

6-33 *(A)* and *(B)* The correct position of the forceps in the posterior half of the disc space.

sheath into the disc space is uncommon, it can cause complications by allowing deeper access into the intervertebral disc. If there is any doubt whatsoever, the relation of the inserted instruments with the disc space should be reviewed radiographically.

When the instruments are properly positioned in the lateral projection, the forceps are seen in the posterior half of the disc space (Fig. 6-33). While in the AP view, the instrument is centrally located. It should be noted that most of the offending nuclear material is located adjacent to the tip of the inserted sheath rather than in the center of the disc space. The straight and curved forceps are introduced, and the disc material adjacent to the open end of the working sheath toward the sight of the herniation is grasped and evacuated. This is followed by the removal of the remainder of the nucleus from the center and the posterior half of the disc. Evacuation of the anterior part of the nuclear material may not be necessary. If deeper access into the intervertebral disc is desirable following the flouroscopic evaluation the working sheath is further advanced into the annulus, and further evacuation is accomplished.

The power-driven instruments (Fig. 6-34) are extremely useful for the extraction of the nuclear material from the center of the intervertebral disc. However, it does not allow access to interannular or subligamentous fragments, and the use of manual instruments becomes mandatory. The high level of negative pressure is introduced into the center of the disc intermittently using a suction pump. This step is followed with further evacuation as described above. The working sheath is engaged and advanced into the annular fibers for a distance of not more than 2 or 3 mm, prior to the introduction of discoscope, powered nuclear resectors and high negative pressure. This simple maneuver establishes a closed suction irrigation system. It is designed to protect the periannular structures while a high negative pressure is introduced or when the powered instruments are being used.

The deflector tube and flexible forceps not only allow access to the posterior half of the intervertebral disc but they are also useful tools for obtaining access to the L5-S1 disc space.

The adequacy of the evacuation of the nuclear material from the posterior part of the interverte-

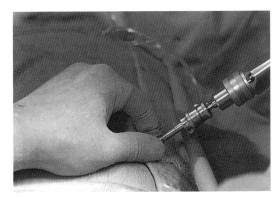

6-34 The powered instrument is shown inside the working sheath and the drop-lock attachment during the surgery.

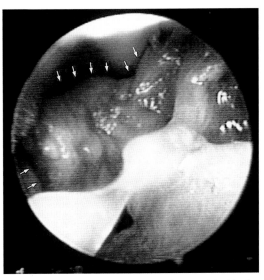

6-36 A free collagenized nucleus fragment inside the disc space as viewed with discoscope.

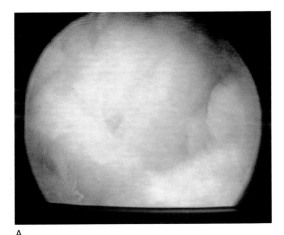

A

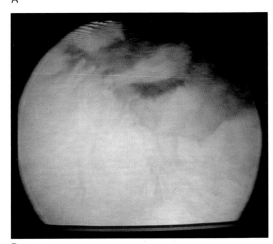

B

6-35 *(A)* Cottonball appearance of the nucleus in a 22-year-old male. *(B)* Partial resection of the annulus with a punch forcep is shown.

bral disc is viewed periodically through the discoscope. An attempt should be made to remove all of the nuclear material which is positioned behind the annulus adjacent to the herniation site. The annulus contains thick, coarse, and whitish fibers which make it distinguishable from the nucleus. In a younger individual the nucleus has a cottonball appearance. It is firm and pliable and is easily cut and removed by forceps or powered instruments (Fig. 6-35). In older intervertebral discs the collagenized nucleus may remain attached or completely detached as a free fragment (internal sequestration, Fig. 6-36).

With the aid of rotary-powered instruments, the site of the annular fenestration is cleaned from the residue of the nuclear material and the debris. This will ensure the continuous decompression following the termination of this operative procedure (Fig. 6-37C).

Prior to the termination of the procedure and the withdrawal of the working sheath a final inspection with the aid of the discoscope is carried out. One should make certain that an adequate cavity or corridor has been created behind the posterior annulus (Fig. 6-37A and B), and the internal semiattached or loose collagenized fragments have been removed.

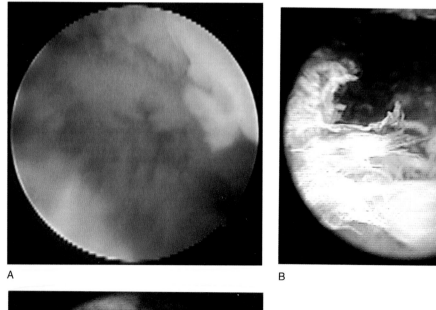

A

B

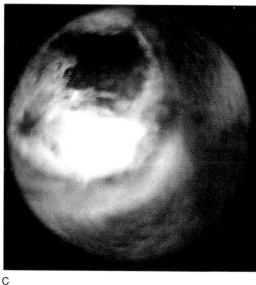

C

6-37 *(A)* Discoscopic appearance of the cavity created behind the annulus as viewed from the inside of the disc space. *(B)* The working sheath is partially withdrawn. Note the thick whitish colored annular fibers adjacent to the distal extremity of the discoscope. The corridor behind the annulus is seen behind the annular fenestration. *(C)* The working sheath is now further withdrawn. The annular fenestration is demonstrated.

Access to L5-S1 Intervertebral Disc

The proper positioning of the patient by keeping the lumbar spine in completely flat or in slight flexion is essential. The weight of the lower extremities may be used for traction by keeping the patient's flexed knees free and away from the bent surface of the operating room table. While the patient is on the adjustable flexion frame on the operating table in prone position, a slight tilt of the pelvis to the opposite side of the entry point further facilitates access to L5-S1 intevertebral disc.

When the iliac spine is rather prominent and the angle between the medial extremity of the iliac crest and the proximal plate of the first sacral segment is acute, one may have no alternative but to select a point of entry closer to the midline to bypass the iliac crest and gain access to the intervertebral disc.

Following the positioning of the working sheath

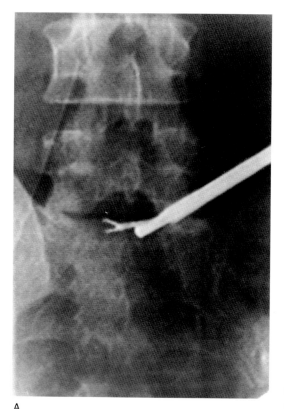

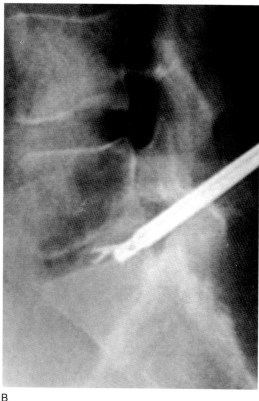

A

B

6-38 *(A)* AP, C-arm view showing the approach to L5-S1 intervertebral disc. The deflector tube allows the deflection of the inserted flexible forceps and fascilitates its entry and evacuation of the disc material at the L5-S1 level. *(B)* The lateral projection of Figure 38 A.

in the routine fashion, the fenestration of the annulus is accomplished with the circular cutter. However, when the iliac crest is unusually high, which necessitates a rather vertical introduction of the instruments, one should not attempt the full insertion of the cutting instrument. In this case the blades may penetrate the proximal plate of the first sacral segment, thus causing undue bleeding.

Following the fenestration of the annulus while the working sheath is held firmly against it, the disc material adjacent to the open end of the working sheath is grasped with the manual instruments and evacuated. At this time the cannulated trocar is reintroduced into the working sheath entering the disc space. The trocar is used as a guide, and the sheath is further advanced into the annulus with firm rotary movement. Usually the sturdiness of the instruments allows a slight separation and tilt between the vertebral plates of L5 and the first sacral segment when they are forced into the disc space. This step is followed by reintroduction of manual and power-driven instruments for further evacuation of the disc material. The deflector tube provides further access to the L5-S1 disc space. As the lower extremity of the deflector tube rests on the proximal plate of the first sacral segment it allows 40 ° of angulation of the inserted flexible forceps and fascilitates its entry into the center of the L5-S1 intervertebral disc (Fig. 6-38).

Postoperative Management

The procedure is performed either on an outpatient basis, or patients may be hospitalized overnight for observation and administration of systemic antibiotics. Following the surgery, all patients are transferred to the recovery room where they are kept under close observation. Their neurological status and vital signs are evaluated and recorded. Special attention is given to any expression of abdominal or excess flank pain. The presence or absence of abdominal tenderness and rigidity are recorded. The patients are permitted to become ambulatory as soon as they have sufficiently recovered from the influence of anesthetics. They are instructed to avoid prolonged sitting for one week. Heavy lifting, constant bending, climbing, and crawling are discouraged during the early postoperative weeks. Mild analgesics for pain relief are provided.

Patients usually receive 1 mg of cephalosporin intravenously prior to the sugery. This is followed by two additional doses given at eight-hour intervals. When patients are allergic to penicillin derivatives, 600 mg of cleocin is administered intravenously at eight-hour intervals as described above. To safeguard against postoperative bleeding the aspirin derivatives and nonsteroidal antiinflammatory medications are not prescribed during the first three to four days of the postoperative period.

Only walking exercises are encouraged during the first week of the postopertive stage. The patients are usually evaluated six or seven days following their discharge from the hospital. At this time their neurological status, the presence or absence of tension signs, and the degree of subjective improvement as conveyed by the patient is assessed and recorded. If the patient still demonstrates pain or residual evidence of root irritation he is instructed to continue with the use of antiinflammatory medications for an additional week or two. During this visit the important role of exercises for overall recovery and rehabilitation is further stressed. The exercise programs are directed toward strengthening of the abdominal and paraspinal muscles as well as overall general fitness of the individual. Approximately seven days following the surgery if the patient has access to a swimming pool, swimming exercises would be of great benefit. It has been our experience that the services of a zealous trainer with a high performance expectation during the early postoperative stages is not necessary and at times can be counterproductive. If it is at all possible, the exercise program should be arranged and tailored as such to be pleasant and joyful for the patient rather than being a chore and act of labor.

When the sciatic pain persists postopertively and tension signs remain positive for a period of six weeks after the posterolateral decompression and discectomy, further salvage procedures such as laminectomy or microlumbar discectomy should be contemplated. Certainly if the neurological status of the patient is worsening an earlier definitive surgical intervention becomes necessary.

It is not unusual to witness the persistence of all or part of the preoperative symptoms following the percutaneous lumbar discectomy. One should resist the temptation of exposing the patient to an early salvage procedure. Invariably with patience, further use of antiinflammatory medications, and a proper exercise program, the remainder of the symptoms will have a tendency to cease.

Postoperative Imaging

A routine postoperative CT or MR imaging is costly and unnecessary. However, in order to study the changes in appearance of the contour and shape of the annulus after both routine discectomy following the laminectomy and percutaneous lumbar discectomy we have performed a number of postoperative CT studies. It was interesting to note that there was no significant change in the shape or size of the annulus of the intervertebral discs with a broad base herniation or annular bulge following either the laminectomy, discectomy, or the PLD procedure.

The cessation or reduction in the intensity of pain in this group of patients may be related to the reduction of hydrostatic pressure of the intervertebral disc and ultimate reduction of the size of the protrusion under external forces and work environment. A similar phenomenon has been observed and reported following chemonuc-leotherapy.

In contrast, when localized herniation with a sudden and abrupt change in the contour of the annulus was present the postoperative CT ap-pearances in all of the laminectomy discectomy group and some of the percutaneous lumbar dis-cectomy patients were quite apparent.

Potential Complications

The incidence of complications has been insig-nificant. In skilled hands the fear of causing neural injury in the course of this operative procedure seems to be unfounded. Although greater care should be exercised when attempting the L5-S1 disc extraction, one should not have difficulty in performing percutaneous discectomy in most in-stances at this level. Since the instruments do not penetrate the disc more than 2 cm the chance of rupturing the anterior annulus and thus entering the abdominal cavity and causing injury to the iliac arteries and veins is slim.

The adherence to a strict sterile technique and the use of prophylactic antibiotics should reduce the risk of infection. Certainly, there does exist the possibility of extrusion of the nuclear fragments through the annular opening outside of the foramina. The site of the annular opening is co-vered with the fibers of the psoas muscles (Fig. 6-18). There appears to be adequate uncontained space at this region which can accommodate these fragments.

The surgeon must make certain that the instru-ments are inserted into the correct level as pre-determined by the imaging studies. One must have access to adequate lateral x-ray imaging. The sacrum is visualized, and the surgical level is chosen counting from sacrum cephalad. If the patient is obese, it may become necessary to expose a lateral x-ray film to ensure that the correct disc space has been selected.

The psoas hematoma is usually caused by bleeding from the muscle layers, periannual veins, or when part of the vertebral plate or osteophytes has been severed by the circular cutting instru-ments. These patients may begin to have pain in the groin and anterior thigh region (24). These

symptoms usually subside with rest and supportive therapy. The infiltration of the muscle layers with Xylocaine-containing epinephrine solution and the occasional use of a hemovac has reduced the incidence of this complication.

Although the recovery from the neurological deficit due to infiltration of local anesthetics around the spinal nerve is eminent, the periannular area should not be injected by Xylocaine solution during the course of percutaneous lumbar discec-tomy. Furthermore, when the spinal nerve is anes-thetized, the patient will not respond to pain stimuli, and there would be a greater chance of neural injury by the inserted instruments.

When the needle and the subsequent instru-ments are properly inserted into the triangular working zone under local anesthesia, the chance of injury to the spinal nerve is remote. The needle testing and discoscopic visualization of the an-nulus, which was described in the previous pages, will ensure the absence of spinal nerve entrap-ment. The iliac arteries and veins are anteriorly located, and the chance of injury to these struc-tures is unlikely. The vertical insertion of the 18-gauge needle and the subsequent instruments with-out adequate flouroscopic control is dangerous and should not be attempted.

When the instruments are introduced through a far lateral approach (7) (Fig. 6-39), they may penetrate the abdominal cavity, thus causing vis-ceral injuries. The site of the entry may be pre-

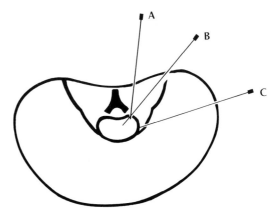

6-39 (A) Incorrect vertical introduction of the needle. (B) Correct position of the needle within the boundary of the muscle fibers. (C) Incorrect horizontal and far lateral introduction of the needle.

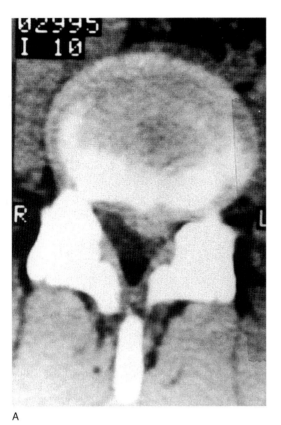

A

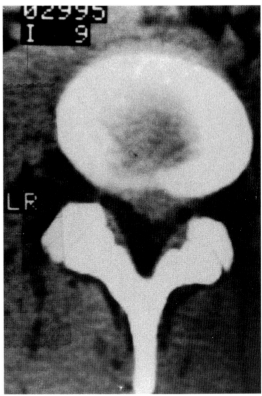

B

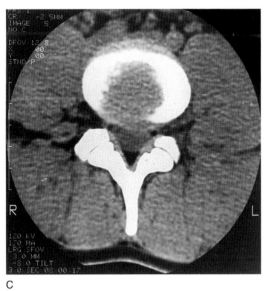

C

6-40 *(A)* and *(B)* The preoperative CT. R.H., 23-year-old weight-lifter with two-year history of low back pain and left sciatica. *(C)* CT scan following posterolateral discectomy and extraction of 2.5 gm of fibrous disc tissue.

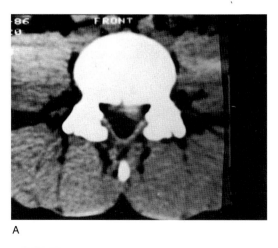

A

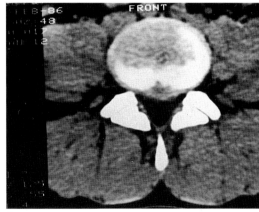

B

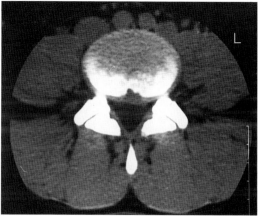

C

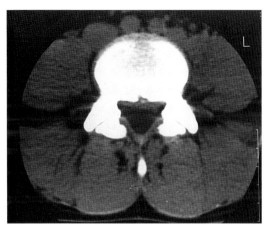

D

6-41 *(A)* and *(B)* The preoperative CT. R.W., a 22-year-old male with 3 months history of low back pain and L5 radiculopathy. *(C)* and *(D)* The postoperative CT demon- strates the reduction of the size of the bulge of the annulus and the evacuation of the subligamentous fragment measured interoperatively 12 × 7 × 3 mm.

determined by a preoperative CT study. In extremely rare occasions a loop of the bowel is found posterior to the psoas muscle which may lay in the path of the inserted instruments. The preoperative CT scan through the herniation site should be reviewed prior to the PLD procedure to prevent such a complication.

The magnetic retrieval is part of the manual instrument set. In the case of instrument breakage it is advisable to use the magnetic retrieval for extraction of the retained piece. The attempt to grab and withdraw the broken instrument with forceps may dislodge it into fibers of the annulus which makes its subsequent retrieval more difficult.

Results

The incidence of failure following posterolateral discectomy in our hands has been relatively low. When patients are properly selected, one can expect up to 85% of satisfactory results following this procedure (25). The most common cause of failure has been the presence of lateral recess stenosis, sequestration, and improper positioning of the instruments which lead to the extraction of the nuclear material from the anterior half of the intervertebral disc rather than the posterior or posterolateral corners. Proper instrument positioning in the triangular working zone is critical to achieve adequate extraction of the above offending nuclear material.

The percutaneous posterolateral discectomy should not be employed only for the treatment of small and insignificant herniations. Rather large disc herniations when proven to be contained may be decompressed and adequately evacuated with the aid of upbiting, flexible forceps and forced suction (Figs. 6-40 and 6-41).

In recent years with the availability of CT and MR imaging surgeons have been diagnosing and treating more patients with foraminal and extraforaminal disc herniations. The evacuation and decompression of the latter through a working sheath inserted just outside of the foramina are accomplished with relative ease and safety (Fig. 6-42).

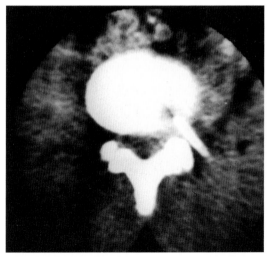

6-42 Interoperative CT showing the inserted instrument entering the herniation site.

References

1. Atken, AP, Bradford, CH: End result of ruptured intervertebral disc in industry. *Am. J. Surg.* 73:365, 1947.
2. Brown, T, Hansen, RJ, Yorra, AJ: Some mechanical tests on the lumbosacral spine with particular reference to the intervertebral disc: A preliminary report. *J. Bone Joint Surg.* 39A:1135, 1957.
3. Collis, JS, Jr, Gardner, WJ: Lumbar discography. An analysis of one thousand cases. *Neurosurgery* 19:452, 1963.
4. Craig, F: Vertebral body biopsy. *J. Bone Joint Surg.* 38:93, 1956.
5. Deburge, A, Benoist, M, Boyer, D: The diagnosis of disc sequestration. *Spine* 9:496, 1984.
6. DePalma, A, Rothman, R: *The Intervertebral Disc.* Philadelphia, W.B. Saunders, 1970.
7. Friedman, W: Percutaneous discectomy: An alternative to chemonucleolysis? *Neurosurgery* 13:542, 1983.
8. Grubb, SA, Lipscomb, HJ, Guilford, WB: The relative value of lumbar roentgenograms, metrizamide myelography and discography in the assessment of patients with chronic low back syndrome. *Spine* 12:281–286, 1987.
9. Hampton, D, Laros, G, MacCarron, R, Franks, D: Healing potential of annulus fibrosis. *Spine,* vol 14, no 4:398–401, 1989.
10. Hausmann, B, Forst, R: Shaving of the lumbar disk space – a new technique in lumbar nucleotomy. *Arch Orthop. Trauma Surg.* 103:284, 1984.
11. Hijikata, S: A method of percutaneous nucleus extraction: A new therapy modality for intervertebral disc herniation. *J. Toden Hosp.* 5:39, 1975.
12. Hijikata, S: Percutaneous nucleotomy: A new concept, technique and 12 years experience. *Clin. Orthop.,* 238:9, 1989.
13. Hiroshi, E: Transverse myelitis following chemonucleolysis. *J. Bone Joint Surg.,* vol 65A, no 9, Dec. 1983.
14. Holt, E: The question of lumbar discography. *J. Bone Joint Surg.* 50:720–726, 1968.
15. Hult, L: Retroperitoneal disc fenestration in low back pain and sciatica. *Acta Orthop. Scand.* 20:342, 1956.
16. Kambin, P: Bulging annulus. *Orthop. Trans.,* vol II, no 1:23 Spring 1987.
17. Kambin, P: Percutaneous lumbar discectomy – safe, effective and cost-efficient. *Orthopaedics Today,* 18, February, 1988.
18. Kambin, P: Percutaneous lumbar discectomy current practice. *Surg. Rounds Orthop.,* Dec. 1988, p 31–35.
19. Kambin, P, Abda, S, Kurpicki, F: Intradiskal pressure and volume recording: Evaluation of normal and abnormal cervical disks. *Clin. Orthop.* 146:144, 1980.
20. Kambin, P, Brager, M: Percutaneous posterolateral discectomy: Anatomy and mechanism. *Clin. Orthop.* 223:145, 1987.
21. Kambin, P, Gellman, H: Percutaneous lateral discectomy of the lumbar spine: A preliminary report. *Clin Orthop.* 174:127, 1983.
22. Kambin, P, Nixon, J, Chait, A, Schaffer, T: Bulging annular protusion pathophysiology and roentgenographic appearance. *Spine* vol 13 no 6:671, 1988.
23. Kambin, P, Sampson, S: Laminectomy versus percutaneous lateral discectomy: A comparative study. *Orthop. Trans.* 8:408, 1984.
24. Kambin, P, Sampson, S: Posterolateral percutaneous suction-excision of herniated lumbar intervertebral discs: Report of interim results. *Clin. Orthop.* 207:37, 1986.
25. Kambin, P, Schaffer, JL: Percutaneous lumbar discectomy – prospective review of 100 patients. *Clin. Orthop.* Jan:24–34, 1989.
26. Lindblom, K: Technique and results in myelography and disc puncture. *ATA Radiol.* 34:321, 1950.
27. Love, JG: Removal of protruded intervertebral discs without laminectomy. *Proc. Staff Meet. Mayo Clin.* 14:800, 1939.
28. MacMillan, J, Kambin, P, Schaffer, JL: Routes of communication of lumbar intervertebral discs with surrounding neural structures. *Spine,* in press, 1989.
29. Markolf, KL, Morris, JM: The structural components of the intervertebral disc. A study of their contributions to the ability of disc to withstand compressive forces. *J. Bone Joint Surg.* 56-A:675–687, 1974.
30. Merriam, WF, Quinnell, RC, Stockdale, HR, Willis, DS: The effect of postural changes in the inferred pressure within the nucleus pulposus during lumbar discography. *Spine* 9:405–408, 1984.
31. Mixter, W, Barr, J: Rupture of intervertebral disc with involvement of the spinal canal. *N. Engl. J. Med.* 211:210, 1934.
32. Monteiro, A: Lateral gap decompression of the lumbar spine. Presented at the international symposium on percutaneous lumbar discectomy, Philadelphia, November 6–7, 1987.
33. Monteiro, A, Lefevre, R, Pieters, G, Wilmet, E: Lateral decompression of a pathological disc in the treatment of lumbar pain and sciatica. *Clin. Orthop.,* 239:56, 1989.

34. Nachemson, A: Lumbar intradiscal pressure. *Acta Orthop. Scand. [Supp.]* 43:104, 1960.

35. Nachemson, A: In vivo discometry in lumbar discs with irregular myelogram. *Acta Orthop. Scand.* 36:418, 1965.

36. O'Brien, JD: The role of fusion for chronic low back pain. *Orthop. Clin. North Am.* 14:1983.

37. Onik, G, Helms, C, Ginsberg, L, Hoaglund, F, Morris, J: Percutaneous lumbar discectomy using a new aspiration probe. *Am. J. Radiol.* 144:1137, 1985.

38. Ritchie, TH, Fahrni, WT: Experimental surgery, age changes in the lumbar intervertebral disc. *Can. J. Surg.* 13:63, 1970.

39. Rydevik, B, Brånemark, PI, Nordborg, G, McLean, WG, Stostrano, J, Fogelberg, M: Effects of chymopapain on nerve tissue. *Spine,* vol 1, no 3:137, 1976.

40. Sachs, BL, Vanharanta, H, Spivey, MA, Guyer, RD, Videman, T, Rashbaum, RF, Johnson, RG, Hochschuler, SH, Mooney, V: Dallas discogram description, a new classification of C-T discography in low back disorders. *Spine,* vol 12, no 3:287, 1987.

41. Sakamoto, T, Yamakawa, H, Tajima, T, Sawaumi, A: A study of percutaneous lumbar nucleotomy and lumbar intradiscal pressure. International. Symposium on percutaneous nucleotomy, Bruxelles, March, 1989.

42. Schreiber, A, Suezawa, Y: Transdiscoscopic percutaneous nucleotomy in disc herniation. *Orthop. Rev.* 15:75, 1986.

43. Schreiber, A, Suezawa, Y, Leu, H: Does percutaneous nucleotomy with discoscopy replace conventional discectomy. Eight years of experience and results in treatment of herniated lumbar disc. *Clin. Orthop.,* no 238, p 35, 1989.

44. Shepperd, JAN:Percutaneous approach to the lumbar spine. Presented at the international symposium on percutaneous lumbar discectomy, Philadelphia, November 6–7, 1987.

45. Shepperd, JAN, James, SE, Leach, AB: Percutaneous disc surgery. *Clin. Orthop.,* 238:43, 1989.

46. Simmons, EG, Segil, CM: An evaluation of discography in localization of symptomatic levels in discogenic disease of the spine. *Clin. Orthop.* 108:69–75, 1975.

47. Smith Laboratories, Inc: *Update on Safety and Efficiency of Chymodiactin,* March 1984.

48. Smith Laboratories, Inc: *Report of Chemonucleolysis Advisory Faculty,* June 1985.

49. Stern, IJ: Biochemistry of chymopapain. *Clin Orthop.* 67:42, 1969.

50. Stern, IJ, Smith, L: Dissolution by chymopapain in vitro of tissue from normal or prolapsed intervertebral disc. *Clin. Orthop.* 50:269, 1967.

51. Suezawa, Y, Jacob, H: Percutaneous nucleotomy. *Arch. Orthop. Trauma Surg.* 105:287, 1986.

52. Suguro, T, Oegema, RT, Bradford, DS: The effects of chymopapain on prolapsed human intervertebral disc: A clinical and correlative histochemical study. *Clin. Orthop.* 213:223, 1986.

53. Virgin, WJ: Experimental investigation into the physical properties of the intervertebral disc. *J. Bone Joint Surg.* 33B:607, 1951.

7 Biportal Percutaneous Lumbar Nucleotomy: Development, Technique and Evolutions

Adam Schreiber and *Hans-Jörg Leu*

Development

Since the clinical introduction of open hemil-aminectomy with posterior discectomy by Mixter and Barr in 1934 (10), a number of specific postoperative problems have been reported. Due to inevitable intraoperative manipulation of the thecal sac in the open posterior approach, the subsequent development of epidural cicatrization is a common problem. Also, the direct dorsal approach across the stabilizing muscles and ligamentary stuctures fosters functional segmental instability. Although the dorsal approach will provide a direct access to the site of a herniation, it may lead to a rather radical discectomy, and, furthermore, with the progression of disc degeneration, the remainder of disc fragments could dislocate toward the epidural space. This may lead to subsequent structural instability and recurrence of radicular pain. Often, the development of so-called postlaminectomy syndrome has to be managed by further neurological decompression, stabilization, or the consideration of another therapeutic concept.

In the diagnostic field, the dorsolateral approach to the vertebral units was described by Ball (1) in 1934, Valls in 1948 (17), and later, in 1956 by Craig (3) and represented the first landmarks in a new direction. The mechanical difficulties with the tools and the restricted quality of available fluoroscopic control prevented the breakthrough and the utilization of the advantageous approach for disc decompression at that time.

Years later, in the early 1970's, Kambin and Gellman (6) applied a modified Craig instrumentarium for posterolateral fenestration of the annulus fibrosis and disc extraction during a classic open laminectomy. By this modification, it was already possible to prevent most epidural scar problems and the reduction of the incidence of

reherniation in the spinal canal. In the same years, Hijikata et al. (4) introduced his own instruments and attempted closed percutaneous removal of herniated disc tissue by a dorsolateral intervertebral puncture.

At our clinic this operative technique was adopted in 1979, using the original Hijikata instruments. It soon became evident that the slim designed instruments conceived for the fine Asiatic build could not completely satisfy the needs of taller European statures. After further anatomical investigations in cooperation with our biomechanical department, we were able to modify the dimensions and design of the cannular system in 1980. The result was a telescope-like pluricannular instrument. After some further modifications in material and finishing, these instruments are still in use (Fig. 7-1). The actual Balgrist cannulas consist of a series of telescopically superimposable and low bendable steel tubes (15). A double-walled guide needle that serves both for contrast discomanometric diagnosis as well as a guide for the introduction of the subsequent cannulas is first utilized. The following overlap cannulas have a conical tip that is not sharpened to cut a cylindrical hole in the annulus fibrosis. So the remainder of the cannulas bluntly penetrate the dorsolateral disc border (Fig. 7-2), thus pushing the annular fibers to the side like an open curtain that can close itself in the weeks following the discharge procedure (9).

In our technique, the natural barrier between the bradytrophic intervertebral disc space and the perivertebral soft tissue can be reestablished. The largest working cannula has an internal diameter of 7 mm and is produced in 10 or 11 cm of length. The sizes of the cannulas are changed in accordance with the variable diameter of soft tissues which require penetration in a given individual during the percutaneous approach.

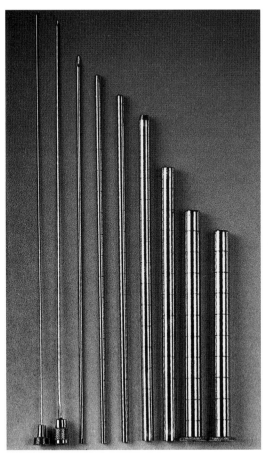

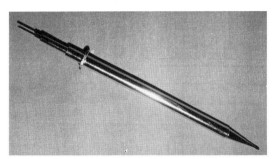

7-2 The tipped ends of the cannulas form a resulting conus that gradually, bluntly penetrates the soft tissues in the percutaneous dorsolateral approach.

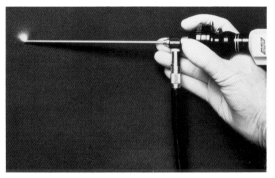

7-1 The Balgrist cannulas for percutaneous nucleotomy with discoscopy (Howmedica®). A set of gradually superimposable cannulas of increasing diameter until 7 mm.

7-3 For discoscopic control a long-shape arthroscopic chip camera with 70° axial deflection and 90° optical aperture is routinely employed.

To obtain more efficient disc decompression we started with a bilateral percutaneous approach in 1981. But even with this modification, we have encountered some difficulties in removing a sufficient amount of subligamental protruded disc tissue. It was impossible to localize the dislodged disc material in the posterior subligamental area. In this event, we attempted to extract the disc material more precisely from the central disc area just to obtain a relative decompression in the dorsal subligamentus zone.

In 1981, preliminary experiments on cadaver specimens in our laboratory demonstrated that the former experimental technique of myeloscopy

(12) could be modified for continuous intradiscal visualization in the course of the bilateral percutaneous approach. In 1982, with an adapted arthroscopic system (Fig. 7-3) we successfully performed, for the first time "in vivo," the percutaneous discoscopy that since has become a helpful routine control of the procedure (Fig. 7-4).

At the same time, the working forceps were gradually redesigned. The rongeurs commonly used in open hemilaminectomy were more effective for extracting loose disc fragments than for picking out degenerative disc tissue. The design of the forceps was further modified to dentated margins and laterally deflected tips. The appropriate

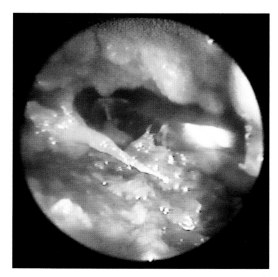

7-4 Typical discoscopic site. The entry of a forceps across the contralateral cannula is directly observed.

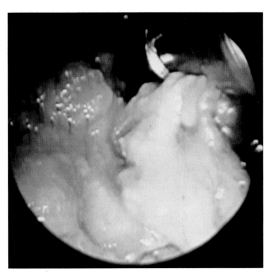

7-6 The disco shaver in action. The optic control looks toward the subligamentar area. The shaver, introduced from the opposite side, gradually devours a major partially mobile disc fragment.

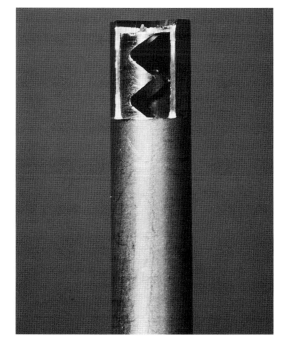

7-5 This 5-mm disco shaver model has a relative large apicolateral abrasive window. The often relative high viscous "mature" disc material needs this larger design in order to avoid tamping.

sizes of forceps were developed to accommodate the various cannulas which are 3 to 7 mm in diameter.

Since 1986, we have employed a motorized shaving device with special working heads adapted to the often higly viscous quality of degenerative disc tissue (Fig. 7-5). This disco shaver works in combination with a high vacuum suction. This system allows the disintegration of the bigger disc fragments under direct discoscopic control before their extraction across the cannulas (Fig. 7-6). It also helps to wash out small particles left behind by the forceps and drains. The optic control irrigation is done from the opposite side via the discoscopy system. The principle of continuous irrigation diminishes the theoretical risk of bacteriological contamination in this bradytrophic area. A routine use of local antibiotics completes the prophylaxis. We do not use local steroid applications at the annular port. In our experience, the disco shaver in combination with the high vacuum aspiration or the respective vacuum punches are appropriate for easy evacuation of disc tissue in younger patients with relatively low discus nucleus pulposus. In patients above 35 years of age, the presence of fibrocartilaginous central disc quality does not permit the sufficient disc extraction in the same way. In these cases, mechanical removal with motorized shaver power or adapted manual forceps under discoscopic control is more effective (Fig. 7-7).

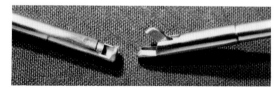

7-7 These long-shaped aspiration punches allow efficacious removal of disc tissue under continuous discoscopic control. The blunt design of the respective tips prevents accidental penetration of the lateral annulus fibrosus at the opposite side of the intervertebral space. As a vacuum source a lipectomy pump is suggested.

Decompressive Indications

The therapeutic spectrum of percutaneous nucleotomy with discoscopy covers today many forms of discogenous low back symptomatology (8, 13, 14, 16). As a general rule, the procedure is appropriate for the treatment of contained (7) disc herniations without free sequestrations. The percutaneous approach may also be adapted in cases where another concomitant lumbar pathology risks further decompensation by open hemilaminectomy. An individual who has had a previous open spine surgery and extensive laminectomy on the adjacent disc and has developed epidural cicatrization may be better served by percutaneous discectomy. In cases where the disc protrusion is associated with posterior instability, such as spondylolysis or minimal spondylolisthesis, we have found particular advantages in percutaneous disc decompression technique. Such treatment preserves the muscular function and allows for rapid rehabilitation and restoration of function, following the surgery. Cases presented with a severe disc degeneration and clinical signs of instability and proven segmental hypermobility by x-ray control will hardly profit from any isolated decompressive intervention without restabilization.

In our experience, the patients selected for percutaneous nucleotomy are of decisive importance (13,14). In addition to the undoubtedly valuable static imaging techniques, functional tests, such as bending myelography and in our later series contrast discomanometry, have markedly contributed to reduce the risk of missed incipient or free sequestrations and preoperative manifestations of degenerative instability.

The Operative Technique

The patient lies in the prone position on a slightly flexed table (10 to 15°) at hip level, in order to compensate lumbar lordosis. The prone position is indispensable for the bilateral percutaneous approach. Another advantage is the lowest possible intradiscal pressure in this position (11). The skin preparation extends as large as 15 cm on each side from the midline. An autoadhesive transparent protection is applied on the skin. The spinal and pelvic landmarks are inked. The level and midline are controlled by fluoroscopy. In cases with marked lordosis, the C-arm is tilted until the intervertebral space is clearly visualized. The entry points are selected 7.5 to 10 cm lateral to the midline and are marked. The distance to the midline can be checked preoperatively in a transparency overlying the preoperatively 1:1 scaled CT scan in the prone position. We try to obtain an angulation to the sagital plane at 45 to 55°. According to the patient's individual stature, this distance may vary (Fig. 7-8). As an anesthetic principle, when no allergic contraindications are present, local anesthesia is recommended. Nevertheless, we have recommended preparation for general anesthesia, such as intravenous perfusion and slight premedication, for every possible eventuality. We use about 5 cc of 1% Xylocaine for infiltration at the marked entry points. To avoid false-negative discomanometric findings due to functionally bicompartmented disc spaces, the first guide needle has to be placed from the side with clinical and radiological alterations (5). Following the introduction of the double-walled guide needle, approximately 5 to 10 cc of local anesthetic are administerel until we reach the level of the transverse processes. The cranial inclination of the fluoroscopy following lumbar lordosis has to be respected also for positioning of the guide needle. At this point, no more instillation should be done in order to avoid radicular anesthesia with loss of pain control. When the patient feels radicular pain, the position of the guide needle has to be moved approximately 3 to 5 mm laterally or medially under fluoroscopic control. A slight lumbar pain is usually felt during the penetration of the annulus fibrosis. The tip of the inner wall of the guide needle ought to be centered one-third ventrally to the dorsal border in the lateral fluoroscopic control while at the midline level in the anteroposterior control. In this position, the contrast discomanometry is performed. Routinely, we use hydrosoluble contrast medium (e. g., Jopamirone®-300, 10 cc) mixed with blue stain (e. g., Indigocarmine, 2 cc). When no discographic-free outflow of contrast medium is visible, discomanometric behavior attests to a contained annulus fibrosis and at least a partial radicular pain ("memory pain") is felt by the patient. In this case, one can proceed with the percutaneous procedure.

In order to have the best control in centering the guide needle from the opposite side, we recommend introducing the second needle as the next step. The radiopaque cannulas will obscure the fluoroscopic visualization of the needle inserted from the opposite side. The second guide needle is introduced in the same way as described for the first one. When the correct position of the needles is achieved, the outside tube of the double-walled needle is kept in situ as a guide, and the inner needle with patent conus, connectable to discomanometric control, is removed. After a small skin incision at the entry points, the stepwise superposition of increasing cannulas over the remaining outer wall can begin. The cannulas are overslipped by continuous rotatory movements. This prevents bending or undue further advancement of the respective inner cannula. The larger calibers are stepwise somewhat shorter so that the smaller caliber inner cannulas can be removed when the correct position of the larger one has been reached.

We recommend to go ahead from the symptomatic side until the third caliber of 3-mm lumen has been introduced. Across this cannula a first decompression with an adapted fine forceps is possible (Fig. 7-9). This helps to prevent further protrusion or even sequestration, due to raised intradiscal pressure caused by the introduction of bigger working cannulas. The same steps are performed from the opposite side. The position of every cannula is periodically controlled by fluoroscopy.

Following the initial decompression from both sides, the larger caliber cannulas are positioned. This final 7-mm cannula has a collar hand stick which facilitates the manual stabilization in the required positon. The tip of this cannula ought to be positioned in the first quarter of the disc space to

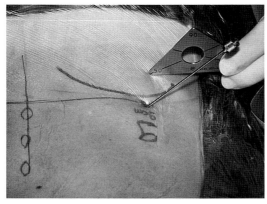

7-8 In this case of a midweight patient, a preoperative CT check enabled us to foresee an entry point of 9 cm lateral to the midline in about 55° sagittal inclination.

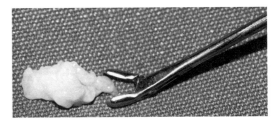

7-9 In the dorsal disc area the disc tissue is drawn out with deflected low-diameter forceps under direct discoscopic control. For patients over 30 years of age the nucleus pulposus is rather a mass of "chewing gum" than the often relatively low viscous "jelly" in young patients under approximately 25 years of age. Here a typical fragment of a relatively matured "chewing gum"-like nucleus is extracted from the subligamentous area.

provide sufficient access to the dorsal subligamentar area. As soon as the working cannulas are positioned from both sides, some nuclear material is extracted with forceps or punches. The aim is to get a first optical space in the dorsal disc area. This can be checked by direct metallic contact between the tools as well as anteroposterior fluoroscopic viewing. A first irrigation has to confirm free flowthrough. Routinely, we use a local antibiotic solution containing neomycin bacitracin, besides an intravenous one dose prophylaxis with cephalosporin. The early irrigation diminishes the stain concentration and allows a better visualization during the following intradiscal illumination.

The review of the preoperative CT scan is helpful in the selection of the appropriate discoscope. In most cases, a deflection of 70 to 90 ° (each with a 90 ° aperture) will be the right choice. Under continuous discoscopic control the disc material from the dorsal subligamentar area is removed. The optic guide allows identification of subligamentary disc fragments, which can be removed without damaging the annulus fibrosis. With adapted shaver models, big fragments can be disintegrated and stepwise extracted. The remaining debris are washed out by the simultaneous suction and irrigation between the discoscope and vacuum punches or disco shaver. In the more central or anterior area of the intervertebral space, we remove just the free disc fragments that could be subjects for later dorsal displacement.

While in the first series we always attempted to take out as much disc material as was possible, following newer biomechanical investigations (2), we have somewhat modified our views. At the present time, we try not to remove more than 3 to 5 gm. As a minimal requirement indicative of sufficient dorsal evacuation, we look for a free optical corridor in the dorsal disc area which is maintained when the cannulas are extracted to the real disc border. This is followed by final abundant irrigation with antibiotic solution. Under such conditions, the cannulas are completely pulled out, and the small skin incisions (1 to 1.5 cm) are sutured with single points or even Steri-Strips® as required.

In narrow intervertebral spaces, especially at L5-S1, the discoscopically controlled procedure has been performed with a 6-mm cannula in combination with the respective smaller working tools.

Discussion

Since our introduction of percutaneous nucleotomy in 1979 and its extension by the introduction of percutaneous discoscopy in 1982, many details have been modified and adapted while the principle of the technique has proven its value. Our clinical experience reveals that the principal advantage of the percutaneous approach has been a rapid restoration of function in 70% of the patients and overall 85% of favorable results. In our experience of over 150 cases, no persistent radicular injury has been encountered as a result of the introduction of an additional portal on the opposite side. The local anesthesia used for the procedure on both sides gives a valuable control. Whenever the introduced guide needle touches the radicular sac, the patient will experience radicular pain. In this case, the repositioning of the needle point is advisable.

References

1. Ball, RD: Needle aspiration biopsy. *J. Tenn. Med. Assoc.* 27:203 1934.
2. Brinckmann, P, Horst M: The influence of vertebral body fracture, intradiscal injection, and partial discectomy on the radial bulge and height of human lumbar discs. *Spine* 10:138–143, 1985.
3. Craig, FS: Vertebral body biopsy. *J. Bone Joint Surg.* 38A:93–95, 1956.
4. Hijikata, S, Yamagishi, M, Nakayama, T, Oomori, K: Percutaneous discectomy: A new treatment method for lumbar disc herniation. *J. Toden Hosp.* 5:5–13, 1975.
5. Ito, S: CT assisted discography. Clinical evaluation of lumbar CT assisted discography in comparison with human cadaver. *J. Jpn. Orthop. Assoc.* 62:345–358, 1988.
6. Kambin, P, Gellman, H: Percutaneous lateral discectomy of the lumbar spine. A preliminary report. *Clin. Orthop.* 174:127–132, 1983.
7. Kambin, P, Nixon, E, Chait, A, Schaffer, JL: Annular protrusion: Pathophysiology and roentgenographic appearance. *Spine* 13:671–675, 1988.
8. Leu, HJ, Schreiber, A: La nucléotomie percutanée avec discoscopie: Expériences depuis 1979 et possibilités aujourd'hui. *Rev. Med. Suisse Romande* 109:477–482, 1989.
9. Markolf, KL, Morris, JM: The structural components of the intervertebral disc. *J. Bone Joint Surg.* 56A:675–687, 1914.
10. Mixter, WJ, Barr, JS: Rupture of the interverteberal disc with involvement of the spinal canal. *N. Engl. J. Med.* 211:210–215, 1934.
11. Nachemson, A, Morris, JM: In vivo measurements of intradiscal pressure. *J. Bone Joint Surg.* 46A:1077–1092, 1964.
12. Ooi, Y, Satoh, Y, Sugawara, S, Mikanagi, K, Morisaki, N: Myeloscopy. *Int. Orthop.* 1:107–111, 1977.
13. Schreiber, A, Suezawa, Y, Leu, HJ: Therapie des Bandscheibenprolaps: Chemonukleolyse versus perkutane Nukleotomie. *Dtsch. Med. Wochenschr.* 113:1482–1485, 1988.
14. Schreiber, A, Suezawa, Y, Leu, HJ: Indication et technique de la nucleotomie percutane avec discoscopie. Evolutions, experiences et resultats entre 1979 et 1987. *Rev. Med. Orthop.* 15:19–23, 1989.
15. Schreiber, A, Suezawa, Y, Leu, HJ: Does percutaneous nucleotomy with discoscopy replace conventional discotomy? *Clin. Orthop.* 238:35–42, 1989.
16. Suezawa, Y, Schreiber, A: Perkutane Nukleotomie mit Diskoskopie: Siebenjährige Erfahrung und Ergebnisse. *Z. Orthop.* 126:1–7, 1988.
17. Valls, J, Ottolenghi, EC, Schajowicz, F: Aspiration biopsy in diagnosis of lesions of vertebral bodies. *J.A.M.A.* 136:376–382, 1948.

8 Automated Percutaneous Discectomy with Nucleotome

Robert G. Watkins

Failure of Percutaneous Discectomy

The percutaneous discectomy is one of the techniques of intradiscal therapy for a disc herniation. It is an indirect method of decreasing the volume of a nucleus pulposus and secondarily decreasing pressure on the herniated portion of the disc. This theoretically decreases nerve root tension. It could remove a contained, herniated fragment, but most postoperative CT scans show it does not. The herniation must have some continuity with the center of the disc in order for the percutaneous nucleotomy to have any effect on the herniation.

Patients with extruded and especially sequestered fragments should not be substantially helped by the percutaneous discectomy. The procedure is best indicated for a contained disc herniation.

Nerve root pain in spinal stenosis is usually caused by a canal, lateral recess or foraminal obstruction due to hard disc bulges and osteophytes. It is possible to have soft disc herniation with stenosis, and a contained disc herniation may be indistinguishable radiographically from a hard asymmetric bulge. Any narrowing of the disc space associated with stenosis may become worse following nucleotomy. Nerve root pain due to spinal stenosis is less likely to be helped by percutaneous discectomy.

Back pain results from a great variety of pathomechanical sources. Doing a percutaneous discectomy for back pain without an identifiable source should have a lower success rate. Because there is a bulge on the CT scan or a degenerated disc on the MRI, it does not necessarily follow that this level is the source of the back pain. Without an identifiable radiculopathy, the spinal level responsible for the back pain is difficult to determine. Discography can be of benefit in determining the spinal level for a back pain, but there are false-positives and false-negatives. If back pain is caused by abnormal biomechanical motion in a segment, removing several grams of nucleus may not affect the biomechanical functioning of that neuromotion segment beneficially. Certainly, more time-tested methods of back rehabilitation, i. e., stretching, strengthening, body mechanics, and aerobic conditioning, should not be neglected in deference to a nucleotomy.

There may be isolated cases of a contained herniation lodged in the annulus producing more back pain than leg pain which could benefit from a percutaneous discectomy. These cases may be difficult to identify. The procedure is probably best indicated for cases of sciatica due to a contained disc herniation unresponsive to nonoperative care.

The automated percutaneous discectomy is a procedure in which a 2-mm sucting-cutting device is inserted percutaneously into an intervertebral disc. The device removes several grams of nuclear material. It appears safe and can be done under local anesthesia in the outpatient department. The overall results indicate an approximate 70% effectiveness. Our review of our failures may help in predicting successful candidates for the procedure.

Case 1

This case is a 39-year-old female with chronic low back pain and occasional left thigh discomfort (Fig 8-1). This patient worked well in the nonoperative program but was unable to decrease her mechanical back pain. She underwent percutaneous discectomy and, postoperatively, had little improvement in her low back pain.

Case 2

This case is a 23-year-old professional football player who presents with a history of five months of low back pain with radiation into the left leg.

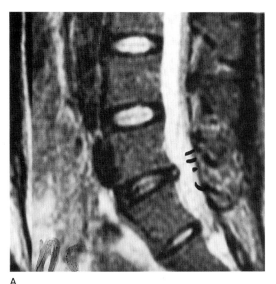 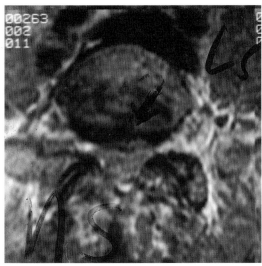

A   B

8-1 (A, B) A 39-year-old female with chronic low back pain underwent automated percutaneous discectomy.

Within 30 days of the onset of back pain he experienced radiating pain into the left lower extremity. Three months after the onset of the pain, it became particularly severe after driving across country. At the time of his presentation, five months later, 100% of his pain was in his left buttocks into the left lower extremity. He had numbness and tingling in his foot for several weeks. On physical examination the patient had a very stiff back with the loss of 75% of lumbar motion and walked with a list to the right. He had ⅘ left gastrocnemius strength and an absent left Achilles reflex. There was decreased sensation on the dorsal and lateral border of the left foot. He had positive straight leg raising, bilaterally worse on the left with a crossover straight leg raise right to left. The Lasègue, flip, bowstring, neck flexion, and foot dorsiflexion tests were positive on the left. Eleven days after presentation the patient underwent percutaneous discectomy. He noticed subjective improvement in his left lower extremity pain for two days, then experienced significant increase in numbness, pain, and inability to spend more than several minutes upright without severe leg pain. He underwent microscopic lumbar discectomy with removal of a large, extruded fragment of intervertebral disc. The patient was dis-

charged four days after admission. Three days after the surgery he began a rehabilitation program and played a full, pain-free season the subsequent year. An additional note in this history – just before the percutaneous discectomy, the EMG showed significant radicular dysfunction, S1 on the left. The impression on the contrast CT scan was soft tissue having disc density extending into the left neuroforamina at the L5-S1 level, compatible with an extruded disc herniation with cephalad migration into the foramina and the lower aspect of the subarticular gutter of L5. The latter may represent a sequestered fragment. There is no evidence of caudal migration.

Case 3

The next patient is a 32-year-old female who presents with a history of four years of low back pain, much worse over the six months prior to presentation (Fig. 8-2). She had a predominantly 70% back pain/30% leg pain problem. The leg pain radiated down both legs to her feet and was worse with walking. She had some tingling in both legs and her feet. Physical examination showed a restricted lumbar range of motion with muscle

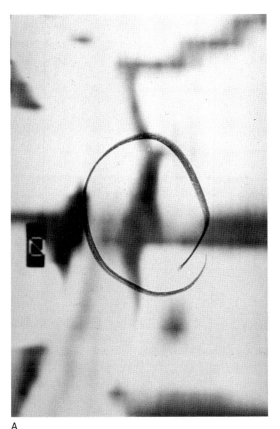

A

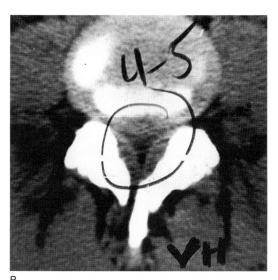

B

8-2 (A, B) A 32-year-old female with a history of low back pain underwent a posterior interbody fusion with back bone and autogenous graft six weeks after the automated percutaneous discectomy.

spasm. She had a positive Lasègue, flip, bowstring, foot dorsiflexion, and neck flexion test bilaterally for leg pain. She also had bilateral sciatic notch tenderness, normal reflexes, bilateral straight leg raising with severe back and buttocks pain. She was treated with epidural injections and a nonoperative back rehabilitation program with an increasing percentage of radiating leg pain. Eight months later she underwent percutaneous discectomy after which she experienced seven days of relief from leg pain. Her leg pain returned much worse in the right leg, but predominantly she had symptoms more compatible with neurogenic claudication than any resting sciatica. She had mildly positive bowstring test and some tenderness in the nerve and positive straight leg rasing at full 90° straight leg raising, but consistent leg pain with walking. Her radicular symptoms increased, and she underwent a posterior interbody fusion with back bone and autogenous graft six weeks after the percutaneous discectomy. Eight weeks after the surgery she had minimal symptomatology and returned to reasonable function. By six months after the surgery she returned to full activities.

Case 4

This 26-year-old male presents with a chief complaint of back pain radiating into the left lower extremity, the onset of which was 9 months prior to visit. The leg pain has become much more severe in the last six weeks. He has sought chiropractic care prior to presentation. His pain is 90% left lower extremity and 10% leg pain, with severe pain while sitting, standing, coughing, and sneezing.

Physical examination on presentation is a 3-cm calf atrophy on the left with positive Lasègue, flip, bowstring foot dorsiflexion test, tenderness in the sciatic notch, and a positive contralateral straight leg raise right to left, positive straight leg raise sitting and supine of the left side.

X-ray evaluation:

There was no documented sensory loss. The patient did have weakness with plantar flexion on the left side.

The patient was treated nonoperatively with an intensive back rehabilitation program and two epidural injections that failed to produce sufficient results. MRI was read as an enormous central and left-sided disc herniation with posterior displacement of the S1 root. The patient underwent a percutaneous discectomy. Postpercutaneous discectomy the patient had relief of his calf pain and was significantly improved for approximately ten days. Then he underwent a complete relapse of severe pain in his leg. A microscopic lumbar discectomy with excision of extruded fragment of intervertebral disc was performed two weeks later. Postoperatively the patient has had a minimum of back and leg symptoms.

Case 5

A 50-year-old private investigator presents with a long history of mechanical back pain treated by chiropractic care (Fig. 8-3). He was initially begun on a back rehabilitation program but returned eight months later with significant back and leg pain. His percentage of back pain was 80% back/20% leg. He did have positive straight leg raising with no neurological deficit in the left leg.

Eleven months after the initial visit the patient underwent percutaneous discectomy at L4-L5. Thirty days postoperatively the patient had no leg pain or straight leg raising but continued back problems. The patient has undergone significant recurrences of back pain in the postoperative period. Nine months postoperatevely he was readmitted with a severe mechanical back dysfunction but did not have recurrence of his leg pain symptoms.

Case 6

This 30-year-old male presents with a history of four years of recurrent back and leg pain treated by physical therapy, chiropractic care, and various nonoperative modalities (Fig. 8-4). One hundred percent of his problem was radiating into his left leg. His physical examination showed 1 cm of left calf atrophy, positive Lasègue, flip, bowstring, dorsiflexion test, positive sacroiliac joint tender-

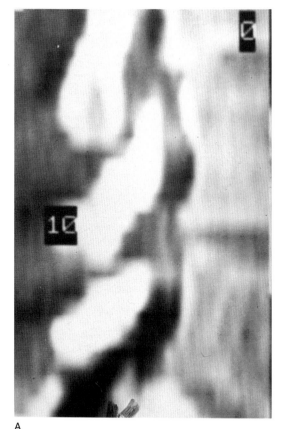

A

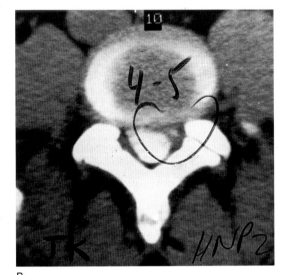

B

8-3 (A, B)   A 50-year-old male with a history of mechanical back pain and sciatica underwent automated percutaneous discectomy at L4-L5. Patient had relief from leg pain but significant back pain persisted.

ness, positive sitting and supine straight leg raise, and a positive contralateral right to left straight leg raise.

Preoperative EMG was abnormal with a left L5 radiculopathy. The preoperative CT scan had a central to left-sided disc herniation, L4-L5 extending into the left lateral recess. Preoperative myelogram was read as a probable inferior migration below the L4-L5 disc space, nonfilling left 5th root. The patient underwent a percutaneous discectomy. Postinjection the patient had no leg pain for two months. After two months he began having vague leg symptoms. He returned to work five months postoperatively. By one year postoperatively he had a slightly positive straight leg raise and pain in his leg. Two and one half years postoperatively he had a flare-up of leg pain and underwent a contrast CT scan that was read as a questionable disc herniation at L4-L5. He was felt not to have sufficient symptoms to warrant surgery and continued to work full time. The EMG two and one half years postoperatively was positive for an L5 radiculopathy.

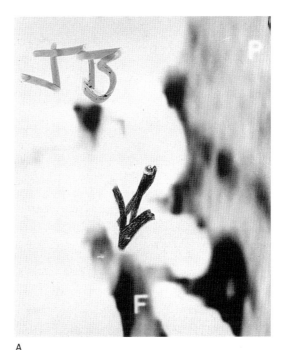

A

Case 7

17-year-old male presents with a history of three months of lower back pain. The pain developed while playing soccer and radiated into the right lower extremity. Two weeks prior to admission, his pain was located solely in the leg. His physical examination showed an absent Achilles reflex and decreased patellar reflex, positive straight leg raising, and a positive contralateral straight leg raise of 60°. His straight leg raising on the involved side was positive 30°. A nonoperative treatment plan was begun with rest, gradually progressing into a spine rehabilitation program. While showing some grandual improvement the patient had a significant relapse three months postpresentation. X-rays at that time revealed a moderate central and left-sided herniation at L4-L5 with moderate central herniation at L3-L4. Three and one half months postvisit the patient underwent a percutaneous discectomy. The patient continued with severe leg pain and a positive crossover straight leg raise and three weeks later underwent a microscopic lumbar discectomy at L3-L4 and L4-L5.

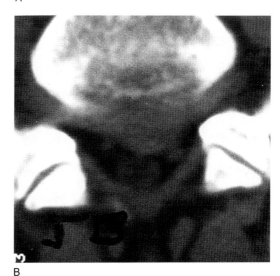

B

8-4 (A, B) A 30-year-old male with recurrent back and leg pain underwent automated percutaneous discectomy. Patient had recurrence of symptoms but was not treated with further surgery.

Postoperatively the patient's sciatica was gone. He still had a very unusual gait and back stiffness that slowly resolved over a two-month period. The patient has had no subsequent leg pain or back symptoms.

Case 8

CM is a 42-year-old male who presents with a chief complaint of back and left leg radiating pain which began nine months prior to his initial office visit. The patient had 50% back and 50% leg pain. The leg pain was increased with coughing and sneezing. At the time of his initial presentation he had positive pain radiation into the thigh, calf, and big toe. He had a positive Lasègue, foot dorsiflexion test, neck flexion test, and positive sitting straight leg raise. The patient was begun on a nonoperative care program and made excellent progress until eight months after the initial visit. The patient experienced a severe increase in numbness in the big toe, leg pain, and positive straight leg raising. At that time the patient had a contrast CT scan that was read as a large central and left-sided disc herniation at L4-L5 extending below the disc space. (Note: At the time of his initial visit the patient had a CT scan that showed a large left L4-L5 disc herniation). Nine months after the initial visit the patient underwent a percutaneous discectomy. The patient experienced an initial total relief of leg pain and big toe paresthesia. Two months postoperatively he developed buttocks pain on the left side. The buttocks pain continued, and seven months after a percutaneous discectomy the patient developed distinctly positive straight leg raising, a weak toe extensor, decreased Achilles reflex, and underwent a microscopic lumbar discectomy. Postoperatively the patient has had excellent symptomatic improvement.

SECTION V
PERCUTANEOUS LUMBAR INTERBODY FUSION

9 Posterolateral Percutaneous Lumbar Interbody Fusion

Parviz Kambin

The detailed description of the anatomy of the spinal nerve and the periannular structures, as well as the radiographic landmarks for the introduction of relatively large instruments, has led us to explore the possibilities of employment of the percutaneous approach to achieve interbody lumbar fusion.

The purpose of this chapter is to familiarize the readers with the work and progress that have been made in the field of percutaneous lumbar interbody fusion. However, at this state of the art, the procedure still is experimental, and its utilization on a routine basis should be discouraged.

The term segmental instability is often used as an indication for spinal fusion. The instability is described by Pope and Panjabi (13) as "a mechanical entity and an unstable structure is one that is not in an optimal state of equilibrium." White and Panjabi (18) have provided a better definition of clinical instability. "Clinical instability is defined as a loss of the ability of the spine under physiologic loads to maintain relationships between vertebrae in such a way that there is neither damage nor subsequent irritation to the spinal cord or nerve roots and in addition, there is no development of incapacitating deformity or pain from structural changes."

There are various kinds of segmental instabilities. Frymoyer and Selby (8) have classified the various instabilities as axial, rotational, translational, retrolisthetic, and postsurgical, the discussion of which is not within the scope of this chapter.

Basically, there has been no uniform consensus among surgeons on the indications for spine fusion. No generally accepted criteria have been developed or published on this subject. The following criteria, which have been described in the literature, appear to be arbitrary and subjective. This includes "prolapsed intervertebral disc in a young patient who wishes to return to the same type of manual work," "prolapsed intervertebral disc with disc space narrowing," "primary central disc herniation," "disc herniation with a long standing history of back pain," and "back pain greater than leg pain."

Although this information is useful in the decision-making process of whether to fuse or not to fuse a given motion segment, it does not represent an objective assessment of the source of pain and disability, nor does it ensure that the patient will indeed benefit from the arthrodesis.

In the clinical arena, the surgical stabilization of a motion segment is justified under the following set of circumstances:

1. When the integrity of the stabilizing structures of the motion segment has been compromised. This includes the developmental instability and defect in the pars interarticularis, surgically induced instability, and posttraumatic fracture or ligamentous injury and subsequent infection.

2. When the ability of the intervertebral disc to contain and transmit the external forces has been altered. This category includes localized degenerative disc disease, associated with facet arthritis and degenerative spondylolisthesis or retrolisthesis, and demonstrable radiographic evidence of hypermobility in the lateral flexion and extension or AP side bending films, and finally, the symptom-producing adult scoliotic curves.

Various operative techniques, namely, posterior (1, 2, 9), posterolateral (17, 20), and posterior interbody fusions (4, 6, 10, 19) and anterior interbody fusions (3, 5, 7, 12, 14, 15), have been utilized for stabilization of the lumbar segments, the discussion of which is not within the scope of this publication.

At times when a mechanically sound operative procedure for stabilization of a motion segment has been carried out for a poor indication, the operative technique has been criticized for

117

the ultimate failure and the unsatisfactory end result.

In recent years, a high rate of satisfactory rigid fusion has been encountered with pedicle screw and plate fixation (11, 16) combined with interbody or posterolateral bone grafting. Despite the radiographic evidence of stability, many of these patients have continued to exhibit pain and have remained disabled.

Certainly, the surgical skill of the surgeon in performing a particular type of segmental fusion, his preference and judgement in selecting the correct operative procedure for a good reason in the right person are the keys to a successful outcome.

The biomechanical advantages of interbody fusion have been well-documented in the literature. The wide surface of bone contact, adequacy of the blood supply, and the natural exposure of the bone grafts to the compression forces are important elements in the success of interbody fusion.

The percutaneous interbody fusion contributes certain advantages and also presents some disadvantages over the conventional anterior or posterior interbody fusion. The posterolateral percutaneous interbody fusion is less invasive and causes minimal injury to the musculoligamentous structures. It leads to a rapid restoration of function and rehabilitation. The procedure does not invade the spinal canal, which is particularly desirable in an individual who had previous spinal surgery and demonstrates severe epidural and perineural fibrosis. However, when surgical decompression of the spine is desirable, this procedure poses a disadvantage.

When the percutaneous route is used to facilitate interbody arthrodesis, the segments are fused in situ. The reduction of a displaced segment or restoration of the height of a narrowed intervertebral disc is not possible without the utilization of external skeletal fixators or interbody expansion devices.

The use of such devices to maintain the height of the intervertebral disc is experimental. Whether or not the vertebral plates will withstand the compression forces remains to be seen. Although the posterior or posteromedial approach with or without laminectomy provides ample space for the introduction of an adequately sized bone graft, the

dimensions of the grafts introduced dorsolaterally through the working sheath are limited to a maximum of 9 to 10 mm.

Operative Technique

The procedure is performed with the patient in a prone position on a radiolucent frame and table (Fig. 9-1). The introduction of the needle and subsequent instruments has been described in Chapter 6. A series of larger working cannulas, which fit snugly over the inserted standard sheath,

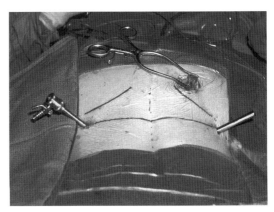

9-1 Intraoperative photo showing two working sheaths introduced into the disc space from a distance of 10 cm from the midline. The self-retainer retractor is placed at the donor site over the posterior superior disc space.

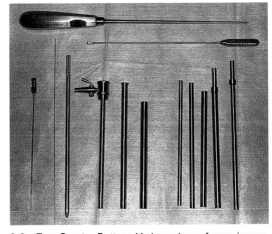

9-2 *Top:* Curets. *Bottom:* Various sizes of superimposable working sheaths and cutting end instruments.

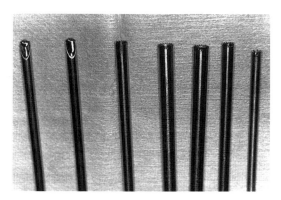

9-3 *Left:* Powered reamers. *Right:* Close-up view of cutting end instruments.

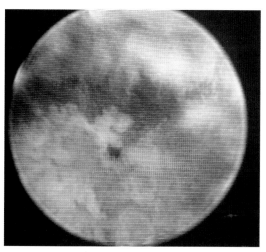

9-5 Discoscopic appearance of the vertebral plate prior to further decortication.

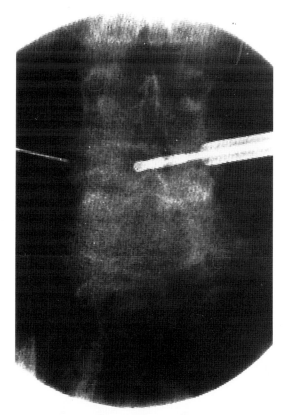

9-4 Intraoperative AP x-ray projection demonstrating that the proper positioning of the needle on the opposite side has been established prior to the introduction of the working sheath and the instruments.

are used to widen the disc space and gain better access to the fusion site (Fig. 9-2). Prototype-powered reamers and various cutting end instruments are employed for the decortication of the vertebral plates (Fig. 9-3). The biportal approach should be utilized. Local anesthesia is used with the anesthesiologist standing by. Prior to the introduction of the working sheath from the opposite side, the correct position of both needles in the AP and lateral projections must be established and documented. The inserted large instruments on one side obstruct the visualization of the needle entering the annulus from the opposite side on the lateral projection (Fig. 9-4).

The disc material is evacuated with the aid of forceps and powered instruments. At least part of the annular ring is left intact for the purpose of containment of the grafts. With the aid of a curet, powered discotomy, or reamers, the cartilaginous surface of the end-plate is removed to bleeding bone (Fig. 9-5). To provide stability, the cortex of the vertebra should not be completely destroyed. We have used a mixture of autologous and frozen allograft bone for grafting. The bone chips are carefully packed at the fusion site. The hemovac is left in place postoperatively for about 48 to 72 hours. We have used a simple lumbosacral corset postoperatively and have allowed the patient to

119

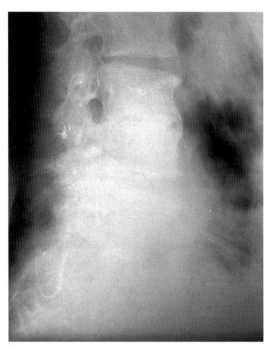

9-6 Successful percutaneous arthrodesis at L3-L4.

become ambulatory shortly following his operative procedure.

Although successful arthrodesis of the lumbar segments by the percutaneous approach is obtainable (Fig. 9-6), our limited experience with short follow-up periods does not allow us to draw a conclusion on the effectiveness of this technique.

References

1. Albee, FH: Transplantation of a portion of the tibia into the spine for Pott's disease. A preliminary report. *J.A.M.A.* 57:855, 1911.
2. Bosworth, DM: Clothespin graft of the spine for spondylolisthesis and laminal defects. *Am. J. Surg.* 67:61, 1945.
3. Capener, N: Spondylolisthesis. *Br. J. Surg.* 19:374, 1932.
4. Cloward, RB: Long-term result of PLIF. In Lin PM (ed.): *Posterior Lumbar Interbody Fusion,* pp 161–164. Springfield, IL, Charles C Thomas 1982.
5. Crock, HV: Anterior lumbar interbody fusion: Indication for its use and notes on surgical technique. *Clin. Orthop.* 165: 1981.
6. Dommisse, GF: Lumbo-sacral interbody spinal fusion. *J. Bone Joint Surg.* 41-B:87, 1959.
7. Freebody, D: Anterior transperitoneal lumbar fusion. *J. Bone Joint Surg.* 58B:193–198, 1976.
8. Frymoyer, JW, Selby, DK: Segmental instability rationale for treatment. *Spine* 10:280, 1985.
9. Hibbs, RA: An operation for Pott's disease of the spine. *J.A.M.A.* 59:433, 1912.
10. Lin, PM, Cautilli, R, Joyce, MF: Posterior lumbar interbody fusion. *Clin. Orthop.* 80:154–168, 1983.
11. Luque, ER: The anatomic basis and development of segmental spinal instrumentation. *Spine* 7:256, 1982.
12. Mercer, W: Spondylolisthesis: With a description of a new method of operative treatment and notes of ten cases. *Edinburgh Med. J.* 43:545, 1936.
13. Pope, MH, Panjabi, MM: Biomechanical definitions of spinal instability. *Spine* 10:254, 1985.
14. Selby, DK, Henderson, RJ, Blumenthal, S, et al: Anterior lumbar fusion, In White AH (ed.): *Lumbar Spine Surgery,* pp. 383–402. C. V. Mosby, St. Louis, 1987.
15. Speed, Kellogg: Spondylolisthesis: Treatment by anterior bone graft. *Arch. Surg.* 37:175, 1938.
16. Steffee, AD, Biscup, RS, Sitkowski, D. J.: Segmental spine plates with pedicle screw fixation: A new internal fixation device for disorders of the lumbar and thoracolumbar spine. *Clin. Orthop.* 203:45, 1986.
17. Watkins, MB: Posterolateral fusion of the lumbar and lumbosacral spine. *J. Bone Joint Surg.* 35-A:1014, 1953.
18. White, A, Panjabi, MM: *Clinical Biomechanics of the Spine.* J.B. Lippincott, Philadelphia, 1978.
19. Wiltberger, R: Intervertebral body fusion by the use of posterior bone dowel. 35:69–79, 1964.
20. Wiltse, LL, Bateman, JG, Hutchinson, RH, Nelson, WE: The paraspinal sacrospinalis-splitting approach to the lumbar spine. *J. Bone Joint Surg.* 50-A:919, 1968.

10 Percutaneous Lumbar Restabilization

Hans-Jörg Leu and *Adam Schreiber*

After ten years of evolutions and clinical experience in percutaneous nucleotomy with discoscopy, there remains the question of whether this approach could also be applied to conditions other than decompressive indications. Soon after the introduction of lumbar laminectomy and disc surgery, the need for vertebral fusion in the treatment of postoperative segmental instability was discussed in early orthopaedic literature (1, 2, 3). This instability may often increase the incidence of peridural scar formation after open hemilaminectomy. In general, the presence of monosegmental degeneration associated with instability and/or dorsal foraminal narrowing above the lumbosacral disc space often creates difficult problems in operative indications.

On one hand the segmental instability calls for surgical stabilization with simultaneous realignment or distraction. On the other hand, the common dorsal procedure even with monosegmental instrumentation undoubtedly weakens the adjacent functional segments. Every open dorsal stabilization requires a more or less invasive approach across the dorsal stabilizing musculoligamentous structures with limited possibility for postoperative muscular recompensation. When it becomes necessary to remove the later implants, the muscular functional compensation will be again impaired.

Unfortunately, modern CT scans and noninvasive MR scans are extremely senitive to metallic implants. Thus, the postoperative evaluation of the stabilizing segment or the adjacent disc spaces with the above modern techniques would be difficult.

For the first time in 1987, we decided to profit from our bilateral percutaneous approach with continuous discoscopic control to develop a technique for intervertebral stabilization (5). The idea at that time was not yet to obtain a solid intervertebral fusion, but just a kind of intervertebral space holder. Following the routinely performed percutaneous nucleotomy from both sides, we implanted autologous bone grafts from the iliac crest. The results were in part not long-lasting due to absorbtion of the autologous space holder in the bradytrophic intervertebral space. With this experience, in 1988 we were looking for possibilities of percutaneous interbody fusion (4, 5). The main problem was to bring enough abrasive power across the cannulas laterally toward the vertebral plates. Obviously, sufficient decortication of the vertebral plates remains a primary condition for solid ingrowth of autologous bone grafts. So, we developed an excentrically guided percutaneous milling cutter (Fig. 10-1) whose action can be visualized by a discoscope introduced from the opposite side.

At the present time, we perform this procedure in two stages. In the first stage, under general anesthesia, the external transpedicular fixators are introduced across the concerned level. The patient is mobilized the same day. The intervertebral alignment and/or distraction can be corrected gradually until the most satisfactory position is achieved. Then, in the second intervention, under intravenous neuroleptic anesthesia, which preserves the patient's response to pain stimulants, still permitting radicular pain to be felt, the cannulas are introduced. A radical percutaneous nucleotomy is performed following the standard steps which were described in Chapter 6. The milling cutter is then introduced (Fig. 10-2). Under direct discoscopic control, the adjacent vertebral plates are decorticated to the bleeding spongiose bone level. For the optic control, the simultaneous irrigation is important to clean up the discoscopic view. The same procedure is performed from the opposite side. With the milling cutter a cylindrically formed bed of at least 14 mm in diameter for the graft can be prepared from both sides. Intermittently the debris is cleaned out under optic control

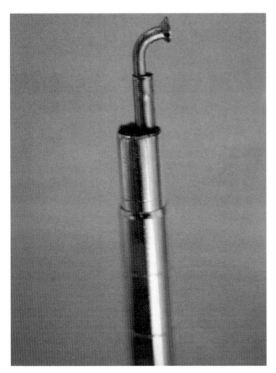

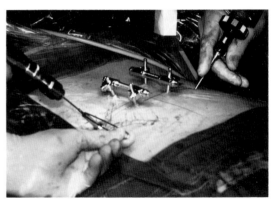

10-2 The milling cutter is acting from the left side, while from the right the discoscopy permanently controls the procedure. The external transpedicular fixator maintains the requested intervertebral position during the procedure.

10-1 The Balgrist milling cutter, introduced across the 7-mm working cannula, brings abrasive power 3 to 4 mm laterally to the cannula so that an open cylindric bed up to 14 mm in diameter can be prepared for later impacted autologous bone. Also, by slight tilting of the working cannula, a deeper opening of the plates is possible if necessary.

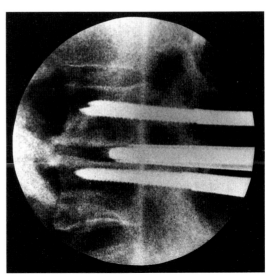

10-3 The intervertebral grafting can be gradually controlled in fluoroscopy until the due fluoroopaque intervertebral plomb is visible.

using the aspiration punch instead of the milling cutter. When sufficient opening of the plates has been verified, the autologous bone from the iliac crest is impacted from both sides across the inserted cannulas. When the optimal impaction of the grafts in the intervertebral disc space is attained (Fig. 10-3) and confirmed by biplane fluoroscopic control, the cannulas are removed. As the cannulas are pulled out, the bluntly penetrated "curtain" of annular fibers may close, thus allowing the containment of the autologous bone grafts. As a final step, the previously distracting external fixators are relaxed, and a slight compression across the fusion site is applied.

The postoperative rehabilitation starts with the patient's mobilization on the first postoperative day with an abdominal support. Three to five days later, a plaster brace with a large window to accommodate the external fixator is applied for two time periods of six weeks. The supervision is continued on an outpatient basis during this period of time. Following the subsequent x-ray evaluation, the two connecting bars are removed. As soon as the patient becomes pain-free with movement and activity, the transpedicular screws are also removed. So usually after three months, free mobilization with controlled physiotherapeutic stabilization is allowed.

This alternative procedure for percutaneous intervertebral stabilization in two stages, as described above, may be performed in part on an outpatient basis. Besides the clinical advantages of the preservation of the muscular stabilizing function and short-term hospitalization, the "bikini-compatible" skin scars, which are hardly visible, may bolster the patient's spirits and personal integrity.

References

1. Briggs, H, Milligan, PR: Cip fusion of the low back following exploration of the spinal canal. *J. Bone Joint Surg.* 26A: 125–130, 1944.
2. Caldwell, GA, Sheppard, WB: Criteria for spinal fusion following removal of a protruded nucleus pulposus. *J. Bone Joint Surg.* 30A:971–980, 1948.
3. Cloward, RB: The treatment of ruptured lumbar disc by vertebral body fusion. Indications, operative technique, after care. *J. Neurosurg.* 10:154, 1953.
4. Leu, HJ, Schreiber, A: La nucleotomie percutanee avec discoscopie: experiences depuis 1979 et possibilites aujourd'hui. *Rev. Med. Suisse Rom.* 109:477–482, 1989.
5. Schreiber, A, Leu, HJ: Restabilisation intervertebrale et arthrodese intersomatique percutanee: Possibilites aujourd'hui. Rachis 1:173–179, 1989.

11 Percutaneous and Minimal Intervention Spinal Fusion

J. A. N. Shepperd

Introduction

As a method of controlling supposed mechanical back pain, arthrodesis of the low lumbar spine has been disappointing. Practical experience over several decades has produced many reports of clinical failure. Three overriding difficulties arise: *(a)* accurate identification of a pain source and confirmation of reversibility; *(b)* achievement of sound fusion; and *(c)* depending on the technique, incidental damage to adjacent anatomy, including posterior primary ramus, theca, ligaments, and muscles. The altered mechanics impose inevitable risk to adjacent segments, and all of this damage in itself is capable of generating pain.

Our center is committed to minimal intervention surgery where possible, and all our procedures are undertaken on a specially developed radiolucent universal spinal table which permits optimal patient position. All procedures rely on x-ray control and are employed for diagnostic and therapeutic purposes, including disc excision and fusion. The approach is either posterolateral or posteromedial.

Diagnostic Spinal Probing

This technique is employed routinely as a method of identifying pain source and confirming that symptoms are reversible. It relies on the establishment of a diagnostic triad, namely, *(a)* an identifiable lesion in the spine is seen; *(b)* when stimulated this lesion produces the patient's symptoms; and *(c)* when a local anesthetic is injected into the structure the symptoms are abolished. The procedure is undertaken with an anesthetist trained in this technique sedating the patient's level of consciousness to one of tolerance but sufficient alertness to respond. It also provides an opportunity to assess the patient's perception and tolerance of

pain. The structures investigated by the probing, which is undertaken with a 1.5-mm trochar and cannula, include the paraspinal muscles, the facet joint, the subfacet perinerve root region, the lateral expansion of the posterior longitudinal ligament overlying the disc, and discography with distension of the disc. The anesthetic agent used in spinal probing is routinely accompanied by a steroid injection targeted into the painful and supposedly inflamed structure. This maneuver alone appears to relieve symptoms in approximately 50% of patients with long-term benefit. Following probing the patient returns to the ward and is invited to mobilize and undertake activities which would normally provoke symptoms and report the effect both in the initial six hours and the subsequent 14 days following probing. Only if symptoms are fully relieved in the six-hour period and revert to the preprobing state over the subsequent two weeks is fusion considered. Close discussion with the patient follows, and it is important to establish that he fully comprehends the nature of the procedure intended.

Posterolateral Access

The conventional 45° posterolateral approach has been studied anatomically. It has been found that provided preoperative probing suggests a straightforward anatomy and that a blunt initial probe is placed into the intervertebral disc in the correct anatomical position, access up to 10 mm is safe at both L4-L5 and L5-S1.

Blind Posteromedial Access

This approach relies again on x-ray control using the special operating table and permits direct visualization of the nerve root in the lateral recess. A 14-mm portal can be obtained.

Procedure

The patient is under general anesthetic, and the appropriate site for the skin incision of 2 cm is identified by placement of a probe in the midline and absolutely parallel with the intervertebral disc of the segment to be fused. The probe is advanced as far as the lower border of the lamina of the upper vertebra. The incision is extended down adjacent to the interspinous ligament, and a 1.5-mm Cobb periosteal elevator develops a plane between the ligament and the muscle down to the ligamentum flavum. The position of the Cobb is confirmed with the image intensifier. A specially developed lever is now placed with x-ray control laterally over the outer margin of the facet joint. Retraction on the lever now permits direct vision of the ligamentum flavum with overhead illumination. A specially developed fiberoptic sucking root retractor provides illuminated and dry visualisation of the lateral recess and nerve root. The disc is identified with x-ray control, and the same coaxial system of tubes is employed as for the posterolateral access.

Percutaneous Fusion

Using the posterolateral access, early attempts at achieving minimal intervention fusion employed homograft bone dowels and fill-in piecemeal grafts. Having established access to the intervertebral disc, thorough excision of disc material was achieved. The bone ends were reamed with a reamer, surplus cartilage curetted with a ring curette, and bilateral oblique grafting dowels were placed. Because of the inability to visualize lateral recess, reestablishment of disc height was intended by using large enough dowels. All patients were discharged from the hospital after 48 hours. Fifteen patients underwent this procedure, and follow-up is now two to five years. No complications arose as a result of the approach. Radiological confirmation of interbody fusion has always been a problem. In only six cases was the evidence of fusion thought to be unequivocal. Eight patients had a good result. Loss of the initial disc height correction occurred in 14 of 15. Because of what was considered to be unsatisfactory results, this

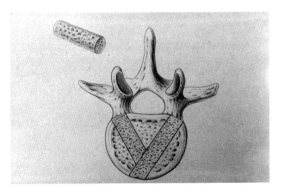

11-1 Percutaneous bone grafting technique employed piecemeal graft and bilateral placement of dowels. The procedure at the present time has been abandoned.

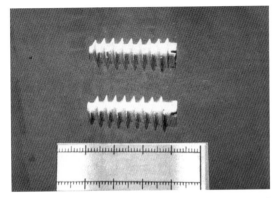

11-2 Spinal bullet. An expansion bullet device is used for both the posteromedial and posterolateral approach.

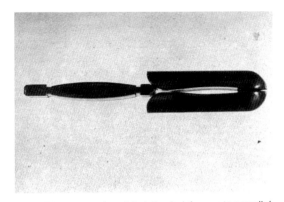

11-3 The screw dowel is intended for posteromedial introduction. The flutes engage the end-plates sufficiently to obviate the risk of retropulsion, although transfacet stapling is also employed. Because of the larger access portal the need for an expansion device is obviated. This device is particularly appropriate at L5/S1.

procedure has now been abandoned (Fig. 11-1). The problem of weakness of bone graft and also the difficulty of obtaining a secure interference fit with a graft which can at best only be the inner diameter of the tube have led us to produce implants. Two implants are currently under evaluation:

1 Spinal bullet. An expansion bullet device (Fig. 11-2) has been developed for both the posteromedial and posterolateral approach. It is intended to be supplemented by a hydroxyapatite and bone marrow slurry. The device may be introduced through a 10-mm portal, but subsequent expansion is possible up to a diameter of 14 mm by the use of the expansion tablet which is advanced after the initial split dowel. The expansion tablet can be provided with two flat ends which lock the position. Posterior fixation using transfacet north-south staples improves stability.

2 Hydroxyapatite screw dowel. Using the posteromedial approach in vitro testing has indicated a risk of instability of the expansion bul-

let. The significance of retropulsion of the bullet is such that we regard this device as unacceptable in this application. We have therefore developed an hydroxyapatite-coated screw dowel (Fig. 11-3).

Future Developments

Cadaver and laboratory studies on the internal disc dynamics suggest that neither disc excision nor spinal arthrodesis is desirable. A healthy disc depends on an appropriate distribution of load between the nucleus and the annulus fibrosis. If the nuclear load is reduced, end-plate pressure produces grinding and thereby destruction of the posterior annulus. In many instances this will lead to further symptomatic damage. We believe that the next phase of enquiry must seek to substitute excised and damaged nuclear material with prosthetic replacements, and we are currently actively involved investigating this area.

SECTION VI
PERCUTANEOUS LASER DISC SURGERY

12   Laser Nuclear Ablation

Parviz Kambin

Although the percutaneous posterolateral discectomy with mechanical tools has proven to be safe and effective, the utilization of the laser light in association with mechanical instruments has opened a new window of opportunity in the treatment of symptom-producing herniated intervertebral discs.

The flexibility and maneuverability of the laser fibers as well as the small diameter of the fibers, are the two major advantages of laser nucleolysis. However, the thermal effect and complications associated with scattered light and the potential injury to the deep structures call for caution and pose certain disadvantages. Furthermore, the laser ablation of the collagenized nuclear fragments may be slow and time-consuming.

At the present time, in the United States basically five major types of lasers are available and are being used in various surgical fields. This includes: CO_2 laser, Nd:YAG (neodymium- yttrium aluminum garnet), argon, KTP (potassium titany phosphate), and ultraviolet lasers. Each laser provides a different color light. CO_2 produces a far infrared and Nd:YAG laser a near infrared laser light, both of which are invisible. KTP has a green laser light, and argon produces a visible blue-green color. The ultraviolet excimer laser produces a sky blue light. The last three lasers are all visible (Fig. 12-1).

The depth of penetration is related to the degree of scatter lights. The CO_2 laser produces a thermal effect and tissue penetration of about 1 mm. KTP and argon vaporize an area of about 2 mm in depth. The thermal effect and laser coagulation of the YAG cover an area of about 4 mm; however, this can be reduced with sapphire contact devices. The limited thermal and soft tissue penetration of the CO_2 laser as well as its high absorbability by water are desirable, and it is an appropriate choice for spine surgery, discolysis, and neurosurgical procedures. However, the CO_2 laser is delivered by rather bulky articulating arms, and its utilization for disc surgery is not practical. The minimal thermal effect and limited scattered photon light energy of KTP and ultraviolet lasers as well as their route of delivery through small fibers make them more desirable for laser nuclear ablation.

The ablation effect of laser on the nucleus pulposus and the annulus has been the subject of several cadaveric and animal studies. Wolgin et al., (1) reported a successful ultraviolet (excimer) ablation of intervertebral discs of fresh cadavers. Takumi Yonezawa and his co-workers (2) have utilized the Nd:YAG laser for vaporization of the nucleus in rabbits and goats using a double lumen needle coated with Teflon for the introduction of the laser fibers. These authors have reported no thermal effect or complications.

In the clinical arena the largest series of laser vaporization and denaturation of the nucleus comes to us from Graz, Austria. Professor Ascher et al. (page 137) have reported approximately 75% satisfactory results following nuclear ablation with a 1320 Nd:YAG laser. He recommended 40 watts ×0.4 seconds × 16 to 34 pulses. The fibers are then advanced further following each exposure for a distance of 1 cm. Schreiber et al. (page 101) from the University of Zurich, have used an ultraviolet wave-guided laser through a biportal posterolateral approach under direct discoscopic visualization. The advantages of photoablation with ultraviolet wave guide lasers are the visibility of the laser beam and the absence of the thermal effect.

At The Graduate Hospital, our clinical research on laser nuclear ablation has been directed toward three objectives:
1. To choose the most effective laser with minimal thermic effect.
2. To take advantage of the flexibility of the laser fibers and reach the posterior and posterolateral corners of the discs under endoscopic control (Fig. 12-2).

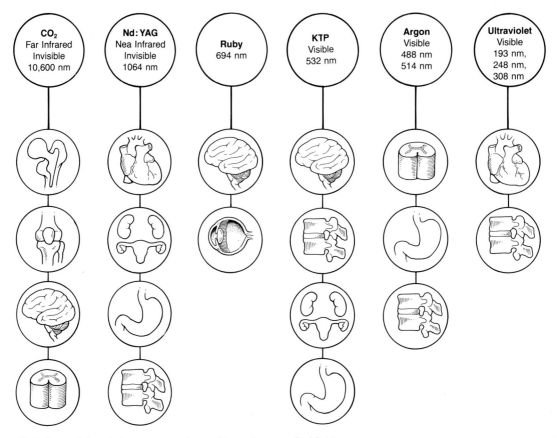

12-1 Laser lights that are commonly used in various surgical fields.

3. To retain the capability of using mechanical instruments in conjunction with laser energy.

We have had both in vivo and in vitro (Fig. 12-3) experience with the Nd:YAG laser. In order to determine the thermal effect of the Nd:YAG laser on neural tissue, we have conducted an in vitro study on fresh cadavers utilizing a cardiac temperature probe. The probe was placed in the posterior longitudinal ligament and the superficial fibers of the posterior annulus. Using 15-watt continuous waves, the nuclear ablation in an area approximately 7 mm from the tip of the temperature probe was conducted for 5.6 seconds. The maximum rise of temperature following the experiment was recorded as 7°F. Intraoperatively, we have measured the thermal effect of the Nd:YAG laser (wavelength 1064 nm) in the periannular region of the intervertebral disc.

A temperature probe was placed on the posterior longitudinal ligament. Using an ER6 Sapphire-tipped probe, the ablation of the nucleus pulposus was carried out. The tip of the probe was placed 1 cm anterior to the posterior longitudinal ligament. Utilizing 25 watts of power for up to 10 seconds of tissue ablation, the temperature on the posterior longitudinal ligament again did not rise more than 7°F (from 90.1°F to 107.1°F).

It should be noted that the length of exposure in these experiments was relatively long; however, in the clinical setting, the rise in tissue temperature was tolerated, and no complications were encountered.

The microscopic examination of the extracted nucleus demonstrated the effect of the laser and was confined to the superficial layers at the site of ablation (Fig. 12-4). The YAG laser should be used with extreme caution during the endoscopic

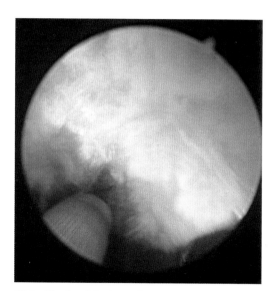

12-2 The tip of the laser fiber is visualized through the uniportal working scope.

disc ablation, where an attempt is being made to reach far posteriorly in order to vaporize the interannular or subligamentous nuclear fragment. We do not have enough data in the literature to pass judgement on the effectiveness and safety of KTP or ultraviolet lasers. The energy which is produced by other commonly used lasers is converted to heat, whereas the action of excimer on tissue is quite different. The ultraviolet breaks the molecular bonds in the process, which is referred to as photomolecular dissociation. There have been two concerns in the clinical use of ultraviolet lasers which included the safety of the gas containers and the possible effect of the excimer laser in altering the DNA structures, which might be carcinogenic. However, it has been reported that 3.8-nm wavelengths are safe, due to the fact that the DNA absorbs less energy at 308 nm than the shorter wavelength excimers. The fact that excimer lasers are athermic makes them desirable for clinic use in disc and spine surgery.

The laser light in combination with computerized tomographic scanning and the stereotaxic system has already been used in neuro and vascular surgery for the aggressive and safe removal of the selected pathologies without causing injury to the surrounding vital cells. This technology opens a new horizon in spine and disc surgery, which certainly is worth pursuing.

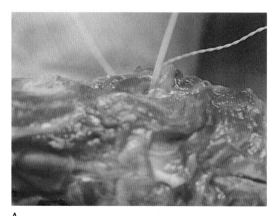

A

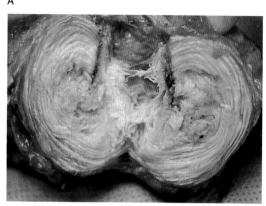

B

12-3 *(A)* In vitro cadaveric study of Nd:YAG nuclear ablation while evaluating its thermic effect on the surrounding tissues. *(B)* Cross-section of the intervertebral disc following laser nuclear ablation with a straight probe. Note the cannulization effect on the nucleus pulposus and annular fibrosis.

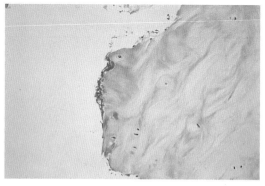

12-4 Microscopic examination following laser nuclear vaporization. Note that the thermal effect was confined to the superficial layers, and the cartilaginous cells adjacent to the site of ablation were not affected.

References

1. Wolgin, M, Finkenberg, J, Papaioannou, T, Segil, C, Soma C., Grundfest W: Excimer ablation of human intervertebral disc at 308 nanometers. *Lasers Surg. Med.* 9:124–131, 1989.

2. Yonezawa, T, Tanka, S, Watanabe, H, Onomura, T, Atsumi, K.: Intradiscal lasar nucleotome. *In International Symposium on Percutaneous Lumbar Discectomy,* Berlin, August 1988.

13 Laser Denaturation of the Nucleus Pulposus of Herniated Intervertebral Discs

Peter W. Ascher, Peter Holzer, Bernd Sutter, Hans Tritthart, and *Oskar Schröttner*

Historical Background

After previous experience with chemonucleolysis in 1980, we performed the first denaturation of the nucleus pulposus (NPD) of a herniated intervertebral disc in 1986. The idea was to decompress the affected nerve by reducing the volume of the herniation. In patients initially treated unsuccessfully with chymopapain and then operated on, we had found dehydrated discs with a tough, asbestos-like texture. If volume could be gained by reducing the water content of the disc, why not vaporize the water? One persisting problem is that the CO_2 laser, which would be ideal since it is completely absorbed in water, cannot be conducted through glass fibers. The neodymium YAG (Nd:YAG) laser with a wavelength of 1.06 nm is poorly absorbed in water, and we expected poor results with its use. Nonetheless, following the suggestion of D.S. Choy, we began in 1986 to denature the nucleus instead of vaporizing it. The first 19 patients underwent the procedure following the introduction of an 18-gauge needle under local anesthesia. All patients reported disappearance of their complaints while on the operating table, but 17 had to undergo conventional surgery within a year because of recurrent pain. Looking to improve energy delivery to the nucleus, we began to use the 1.32 nm Nd:YAG laser. This laser is better absorbed in water than the 1.06 nm model. Studies on cadavers and dogs, done by at our request by H. Jury in Cordoba, Argentina, confirmed our expectations. Twice as much volume was won at the same energy expenditure. We thus began again early in 1988 to perform NPD with the new laser.

Technique

Puncture technique corresponds to the lateral technique described by McCulloch for discography or chymopapain instillation. The physician, nurse, and patient are scrubbed, and sterile precautions are observed. The patient is placed on his or her healthy side, and the point of infiltration is marked about 8 cm lateral to the spinosus process adjacent to the iliac crest (L 4-L5). For the disc L5-S1 the puncture is placed 1 cm caudad and medially (Fig. 13-1). A depot of a local anesthetic agent (we use 1% procaine or lidocaine) can be placed at the nerve of Luschka. The puncture is placed under the vertebral arch and directed towards the articular process. The needle is passed just laterally to the articular process directed to the disc. We use puncture needles developed for us by Aesculap. The needle is aimed at the nucleus pulposus. The resistance of the annulus fibrosus and the passage of the needle through it are easily felt.

The position of the tip of the needle is verified under fluoroscopic control in two planes, and the trochar pulled out (Figs. 13-2 and 13-3). The necessary length of the glass fiber for the 1.32-nm Nd:YAG laser is measured and the 400 nm in diameter laser probe inserted into the needle after

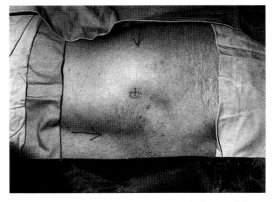

13-1 For the disc L5/S1 the puncture is inserted 1 cm caudal and medially.

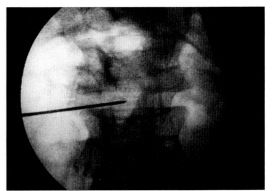

13-3 The position of the needle in the AP plane.

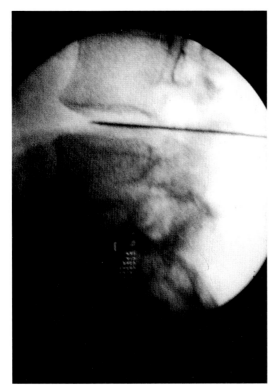

13-2 The position of the tip of the needle is confirmed under fluoroscopic control in the lateral plane.

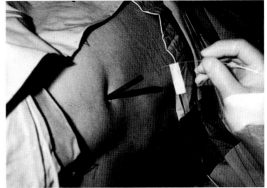

13-4 The glass fiber for the Nd:YAG laser is measured and the laser probe inserted into the needle after it has been marked exactly.

it has been marked exactly (Fig. 13-4). A wide transverse process, moderate to severe osteochondrosis at the articular processes, and obesity can make disc puncture difficult, or, in the segment L5/S1, even impossible. We do not perform a medial puncture because the spinal fluid loss through an 18-gauge needle could cause a low liquid pressure syndrome.

Once the needle has been placed in the nucleus pulposus and its position verified, 1-second single shots of the laser are applied at an average output of 17 to 24 watts at intervals of 1 to 2 mm. The needle is repositioned two or three times and the procedure repeated until 1200 to 1400 joules (J)

have been expended. We generally apply 80 to 110 single shots. The laser time is thus at most 110 seconds. At around 300 J the patients usually spontaneously report that their symptoms are abating. This can be verified by Lasègue's sign. If the patient reports local pain or, less frequently, ischialgiform pain or pain radiating to the lower abdomen, the procedure can be interrupted for a short time to relieve symptoms of high pressure caused by vapor and smoke. The patient leaves the operating table himself and can be discharged from the hospital with a Tigges bandage on the same day. We have performed the procedure on an outpatient basis in a few patients.

Indications

The classic indications for surgery or for chymopapain injection also apply to NPD.

1. Monoradicular compression symptoms (decreased reflexes, motor deficits, segmental pain distribution, Lasègue's sign, Naffziger's sign).
2. Classic protrusion findings by computed tomography (CT) or magnetic resonance imaging (MRI), or by myeolography or discography. We consider medial or mediolateral protrusions ideal for NPD.
3. At least two months of neurological symptoms and conservative treatment. Patients who initially responded well to chirotherapy or blockade but who have recurrent pain are good candidates for NPD.

Approximately half of the 210 patients who have undergone NPD at our department fall into the last group. The remaining patients underwent the procedure because it is well tolerated and complications are rare. We consider NPD the last conservative measure in the treatment of ischialgiform pain in poor-risk patients, unclear cases, and in the presence of what we call a social indication (patients who have filed claims for disability insurance).

To date 210 patients have undergone NPD at our department; 197 (115 men, 82 women) have undergone a follow-up examination (Table 13-1). Sixty four patients reported pain, but 14 were neurologically so much improved that no further treatment was required. Fifty patients were advised to undergo surgery. In about half of these patients surgery revealed classic findings, such as partial sequestrums, lateral adhesions, protrusions, and narrow root canals. These patients were subsequently free of symptoms. The remaining patients showed none of these typical findings and reported continuing ischialgiform or atypical lumbar pain. If it has not been done earlier, the patient's social and psychiatric situation should be evaluated at this point.

Clinical course

Most patients reported alleviation of their symptoms after an energy expenditure of about 300 J while still on the operating table. Improvement can be verified by Lasègue's sign. The patient can get off the operating table on his or her own and can leave the hospital with a fitted lumbar support bandage (Tigges bandage). The patient is told that increased lumbar pain may occur for 4 to 8 weeks. This pain is managed only by decreased physical acitivity and wearing of the Tigges bandage. At 10 to 14 days, most neurological deficits have improved. The restitution time corresponds to the degree and duration of the initial complaints.

Six weeks after NPD, conventional radiography shows a decreased height of the intervertebral

Table 13-1   Segmental Distribution of the NPD Procedure
h8l9m15.6f31

	Right	Left	Total
L2 / L3	1	0	1
L3 / L4	4	7	11
L4 / L5	57	71	129
L5 / L6	7	5	12
L5 / S1	23	22	45
	92	105	197

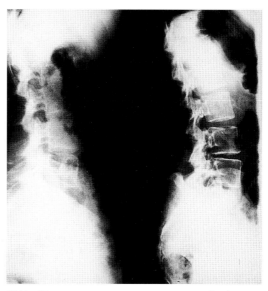

13-5   Six weeks after NPD, the radiograph shows a decreased height of the intervertebral disc.

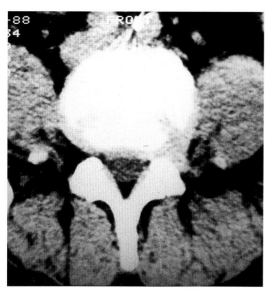 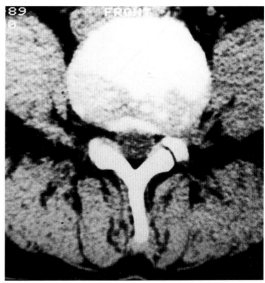

13-6 CT findings regress slowly.

13-7 Air spaces are sometimes seen on the CT scan.

disc (Fig. 13-5). Surprisingly, CT findings regress slowly or not at all. Air spaces are sometimes seen (Figs. 13-6 and 13-7). MR shows a decreased water content of the disc.

One of our 210 patients developed discitis, but retrospectively we could not determine whether a latent process was activated or the infection was introduced by the procedure. We now perform NPD in the operating room under sterile conditions (scrubbing, draping). Preoperative studies include blood counts, erythrocyte sedimentation rate, and, if indicated, scintigraphy.

Discussion

Results of NPD are promising, although the 1.32 nm Nd:YAG is not the ideal laser for the procedure. Approximately 75% of the patients undergoing NPD report continuing relief and need not undergo conventional surgery. New wavelengths or other lasers (for example the 1.44 µm Nd:YAG, Er:YAG, or CO_2 lasers) should provide a breakthrough and offer an alternative to all other percutaneous disc treatments and to surgical volume reduction.

14 Laser Nuclear Photoablation

Hans-Jörg Leu and *Adam Schreiber*

The laser nuclear ablation opens new possibilities in the field of percutaneous nucleotomy. While all thermic lasers, such as CO_2, neodymium, and other types, find their limits for undesirable thermic side effects, the nearly athermic ultraviolet Excimer™ laser, which is conductable in flexible glass fibers, could resolve the often limiting mechanical tool design problems. Our respective first experience in early 1989 has proven the real practicability of excimer laser energy in percutaneous nucleotomy with simultaneous continuous discoscopic control via the biportal approach (Figs. 14-1 and 14-2). With further development of technical specification of more flexible bounded glass fibers and improvement in the Excimer laser's performance, let us expect a larger application of this technique in coming years. With the availability of the flexible fiberoptic, there may be a possibility of continuous discoscopic control of laser photoablative discharges through a uniportal percutaneous approach.

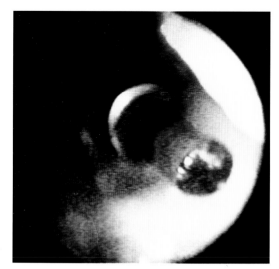

14-1 Excimer laser's 1 mm glass fiber in direct discoscopic control.

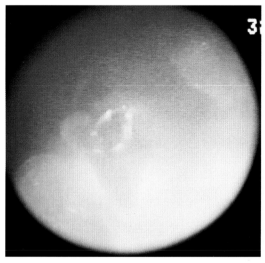

14-2 During photoablation by laser energy the sky blue light of the ultraviolet laser (309-nm) can be followed and directed under discoscopic control *(right)*.

INDEX